Created by Xspurts.com

All rights reserved.

Copyright © 2005 onwards .

By reading this book, you agree to the below Terms and Conditions.

Xspurts.com retains all rights to these products.

No part of this book may be reproduced in any form, by photostat, microfilm, xerography, or any other means, or incorporated into any information retrieval system, electronic or mechanical, without the written permission of Xspurts.com; exceptions are made for brief excerpts used in published reviews.

This publication is designed to provide accurate and authoritative information with regard to the subject matter covered but is for entertainment purposes only. It is sold with the understanding that the publisher is not engaged in rendering legal, accounting, health, relationship or other professional / personal advice. If legal advice or other expert assistance is required, the services of a competent professional should be sought.

♥ A New Zealand Designed Product

Get A Free Book At: https://free.xspurts.com

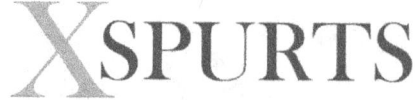

Table of Contents:

Table of Contents:
Understanding Aromatherapy
The History of Aromatherapy
The Basics of Aromatherapy
Differences Between Essential Oils and Fragrances
Essential Oils: The Heart of Aromatherapy
Identifying High-Quality Essential Oils
Understanding the Different Types of Essential Oils
Blending Essential Oils
The Science Behind Aromatherapy
How Aromatherapy Affects the Brain
Physical Effects of Aromatherapy
Safety Precautions and Guidelines
Using Essential Oils Safely
Potential Risks and How to Avoid Them
Using Aromatherapy for Stress Management
Understanding How Stress Affects the Body
Which Essential Oils Are Best for Stress Relief
Essential Oils for Health and Wellness
Boosting the Immune System With Essential Oils
Essential Oils for Pain Management
Improving Sleep Quality Through Aromatherapy
Aromatherapy for Emotional Balancing
Essential Oils for Anxiety and Depression
Aromatherapy for Emotional Wellbeing
Aromatherapy for Skin Care
Essential oils for Different Skin Types
Creating a Natural Skincare Routine with Essential Oils

Aromatherapy for Hair and Scalp Health
Essential oils beneficial for hair and scalp
Crafting Haircare Products with Essential Oils
Creating an Aromatherapy Massage at Home
Selecting the Right Carrier Oils
Techniques for a Relaxing Aromatherapy Massage
Aromatherapy for Mindfulness and Meditation
Choosing Essential Oils for Meditation
Learning to Use Aromatherapy in Your Practice
Aromatherapy in Your Daily Routine
Simple Ways to Incorporate Aromatherapy into your Life
Making Your Own Aromatherapy Products
Exploring Advanced Aromatherapy Techniques
Understanding the Chakras and Aromatherapy
Aromatherapy Reflexology
Expanding Your Aromatherapy Knowledge
Resources for Continuous Learning
Building a Career in Aromatherapy
Have Questions / Comments?
Get Another Book Free

Understanding Aromatherapy

Aromatherapy is a practice that utilizes the natural extracts of plants, commonly known as essential oils, to promote physical and emotional well-being. These oils are derived from flowers, herbs, spices, and other plant materials through processes like distillation or cold pressing. The idea is that the compounds within the essential oils can have therapeutic effects when absorbed into the body through inhalation or topical application, offering a holistic approach to health.

The key to aromatherapy lies in the power of scent. The olfactory system, responsible for our sense of smell, is directly linked to the limbic system in the brain, which governs emotions, memory, and certain physiological functions. This connection explains why inhaling certain fragrances can evoke emotional responses or even trigger memories, while others may help reduce anxiety, promote relaxation, or enhance focus. Essential oils such as lavender, peppermint, and eucalyptus are commonly used for their calming, invigorating, or decongestant properties, respectively.

Aside from its emotional benefits, aromatherapy has been studied for its physical effects on the body. For example, lavender is known for its soothing properties, often used to alleviate stress and promote sleep. Peppermint oil can help relieve tension headaches, and eucalyptus is frequently employed to assist with respiratory issues by opening airways and easing congestion. Tea tree oil, another popular essential oil, is often applied to the skin for its antibacterial and antifungal qualities.

Aromatherapy can be practiced in various ways. Diffusers are commonly used to disperse essential oils into the air, creating an aromatic environment that can influence mood or atmosphere. Topical applications, like in massage oils or skin care products, allow the oils to be absorbed through the skin. Some people may also add essential oils to baths, allowing for both inhalation and skin absorption. The practice is increasingly popular in spas and wellness centers, where it is often used in conjunction with other therapeutic techniques like massage or meditation.

While aromatherapy is generally considered safe when used appropriately, it's important to use essential oils with care. Not all oils are suitable for every individual, and some may cause allergic reactions or skin irritation, especially if used undiluted. Pregnant women, children, and individuals with certain health conditions should exercise caution and consult with a healthcare provider before using essential oils.

The growing interest in aromatherapy is part of a broader trend towards natural and alternative health practices. While more scientific research is needed to fully understand the mechanisms behind its benefits, many people find aromatherapy to be a valuable tool for enhancing mental clarity, relaxation, and overall well-being.

The History of Aromatherapy

The use of plants and their aromatic properties for healing dates back thousands of years, with ancient civilizations recognizing the power of natural oils to promote health and well-being. The history of aromatherapy is intertwined with the development of medicine, religion, and cultural practices, evolving through various eras and regions.

In ancient Egypt, around 4500 BCE, aromatic oils were prized for their therapeutic and cosmetic benefits. Egyptians were among the first to document the use of essential oils in their medical practices, using plant extracts in incense and ointments. They understood the medicinal properties of oils like myrrh and frankincense, which were often used for embalming, religious rituals, and healing. The Ebers Papyrus, an ancient Egyptian medical text dating to around 1500 BCE, lists numerous plant-based remedies, many of which would be considered early forms of aromatherapy.

The Greeks and Romans further advanced the use of aromatic plants. Greek physician Hippocrates, known as the "Father of Medicine," used aromatic oils in his treatments and believed that bathing in fragrant oils had healing powers. Roman soldiers also utilized essential oils for their wounds and injuries. Notably, the Romans were instrumental in popularizing the practice of bathing with essential oils in public baths, a ritual that combined cleanliness with the therapeutic benefits of aromatic plants.

In the Middle Ages, the knowledge of aromatherapy was preserved and expanded by Islamic scholars, many of whom made significant contributions to the field of distillation. Persian physician Avicenna (Ibn Sina), around the 11th century, is credited with the discovery of the process of steam distillation, which allowed for the extraction of essential oils from plants. His work on distillation made it possible to concentrate the healing properties of plants into a more potent and accessible form. This era also saw the widespread use of aromatic herbs like lavender and rosemary in medicine, cooking, and as remedies for a variety of ailments.

During the Renaissance, aromatherapy continued to thrive, particularly in Europe. The use of essential oils as part of herbal medicine gained momentum, with physicians advocating their use for treating everything from digestive issues to infections. In the 16th century, French perfumer and chemist René-Maurice Gattefossé became a key figure in the history of aromatherapy. Gattefossé's accidental discovery of the healing properties of lavender oil when he used it to treat a burn on his hand marked the beginning of modern aromatherapy. He went on to conduct extensive research into the therapeutic properties of essential oils and coined the term "aromatherapy" in the 1930s.

The popularity of aromatherapy grew throughout the 20th century, especially in Europe, as the benefits of essential oils were further explored. In the 1940s, French chemist Jean Valnet expanded on Gattefossé's work, using essential oils in the treatment of wartime injuries and infections. His research solidified the role of essential oils in modern medicine, though they were still considered a complementary form of treatment.

In the 1970s, the practice of aromatherapy began to spread globally, particularly in wellness and alternative health circles. Interest in natural healing and a return to holistic practices fueled the demand for essential oils, and aromatherapy became more widely recognized as a tool for relaxation, stress relief, and emotional balance. Today, it is used in spas, wellness centers, and private homes as an integral part of complementary medicine.

The history of aromatherapy demonstrates a long-standing belief in the power of plants to heal and restore balance to the body and mind. From the ancient Egyptians to modern-day practitioners, the use of essential oils has evolved into a respected and widely practiced holistic treatment that continues to grow in popularity.

The Basics of Aromatherapy

Aromatherapy is a therapeutic practice that utilizes the natural extracts from plants, known as essential oils, to improve physical, mental, and emotional health. These oils are concentrated extracts from flowers, leaves, stems, bark, or roots of various plants and are typically obtained through distillation or cold pressing. The basic principle behind aromatherapy is that these essential oils can influence the body and mind through the sense of smell or by being absorbed into the skin.

The most common method of using essential oils is through inhalation. When inhaled, the molecules of essential oils are detected by the olfactory system, which sends signals directly to the limbic system of the brain—an area responsible for emotions, memory, and some autonomic functions. This connection is why certain scents, such as lavender or eucalyptus, can trigger calming effects, reduce stress, or even enhance focus and clarity. Inhaling essential oils can be done using diffusers, steam inhalations, or simply by breathing in the aroma directly from the bottle.

Another primary method of aromatherapy is topical application, where essential oils are diluted with a carrier oil and massaged into the skin. This approach allows the essential oils to be absorbed into the bloodstream and can be used for a variety of purposes. For example, peppermint oil is often used to relieve headaches or muscle pain, while tea tree oil is known for its antibacterial properties and is commonly used for skin ailments. Always diluting essential oils in a carrier oil, such as coconut, jojoba, or almond oil, is essential to prevent irritation or sensitivity.

Each essential oil has unique properties, and different oils are chosen depending on the desired therapeutic effect. Lavender oil, for instance, is renowned for its ability to promote relaxation and reduce anxiety, making it ideal for stress relief and improving sleep. On the other hand, citrus oils like lemon or orange are uplifting and are often used to boost mood and energy levels. Eucalyptus and peppermint oils are popular choices for respiratory support, helping to clear sinuses or relieve congestion.

While aromatherapy is largely considered safe, it's important to approach it with care. Essential oils are highly concentrated and can cause skin irritation if applied undiluted. Some oils are not recommended for use during pregnancy, for young children, or for individuals with certain health conditions. Always consulting with a qualified professional and performing a patch test before using a new oil can help ensure safety and effectiveness.

The growing interest in aromatherapy has led to its integration into various health and wellness practices, from massage therapy to mindfulness exercises. Whether through its calming effects, its ability to enhance mood, or its support of overall health, aromatherapy continues to be a versatile and natural option for promoting well-being.

Differences Between Essential Oils and Fragrances

Essential oils and fragrances are both widely used in aromatherapy and scent-based products, but they differ significantly in their composition, purpose, and benefits. While they may seem similar in that both provide distinctive scents, the key differences lie in their origin, chemical composition, and how they interact with the body.

Essential oils are natural extracts derived from plants, including flowers, leaves, roots, bark, or seeds, through processes like distillation or cold pressing. These oils contain the plant's aromatic compounds, which are responsible for their distinct fragrances and therapeutic properties. Because they are plant-based, essential oils carry a range of bioactive compounds that can have physiological and emotional effects. For example, lavender oil has calming properties that can help with relaxation and sleep, while eucalyptus oil is known for its respiratory benefits.

Fragrances, on the other hand, are often synthetic mixtures of various chemicals, designed to mimic the scent of natural oils or create entirely new, unique smells. They are used primarily for their aromatic qualities rather than for any therapeutic effects. Fragrance oils can be made from artificial compounds, which means they do not carry the medicinal benefits that essential oils do. These oils are often found in perfumes, candles, air fresheners, and other products intended to enhance the scent of an environment or a personal scent.

One of the major distinctions between essential oils and fragrances is the level of complexity and authenticity. Essential oils contain a broad spectrum of chemical compounds that work in synergy to provide holistic benefits. For instance, the therapeutic effects of peppermint essential oil come from a combination of menthol, menthone, and other compounds, which together help relieve muscle tension or improve focus. Fragrances, however, are typically single, synthetic compounds or a blend of synthetic ones, and do not offer the same multi-dimensional qualities or healing effects.

Another important difference is that essential oils are generally considered safe for topical application and inhalation (when used correctly and in appropriate concentrations), whereas fragrances, due to their synthetic nature, may cause allergic reactions, skin irritation, or other sensitivities in some individuals. Essential oils, when diluted properly, can be massaged into the skin, used in diffusers, or incorporated into bath products for therapeutic benefits. Fragrance oils are typically used in non-therapeutic contexts, and it's advised to avoid applying them directly to the skin unless specifically designed for such use.

Essential oils are also prized in aromatherapy for their emotional and physiological effects. Their use in promoting relaxation, reducing stress, easing pain, or improving mental clarity is rooted in their bioactive components that interact with the body in therapeutic ways. Fragrances, however, are typically used for scent enhancement and ambiance creation without offering medicinal effects.

In conclusion, while both essential oils and fragrances contribute to our sensory experience, they are fundamentally different in terms of origin, chemical composition, and purpose. Essential oils, derived from plants, have therapeutic properties that benefit the body and mind, while fragrances, often synthetic, are primarily designed to produce pleasant scents without any health-related effects. Understanding these differences is important, especially when choosing products for wellness, as essential oils offer far more than just a pleasing aroma.

Essential Oils: The Heart of Aromatherapy

At the core of aromatherapy lies a powerful and versatile tool—essential oils. These concentrated plant extracts have been used for centuries to promote health, enhance mood, and support emotional well-being. Essential oils are derived from various parts of plants, including flowers, leaves, stems, and roots, using processes like steam distillation or cold pressing. Their popularity in aromatherapy stems from their potent therapeutic properties, which can affect both the body and mind in profound ways.

Each essential oil contains a unique blend of chemical compounds that contribute to its distinctive aroma and therapeutic effect. For example, lavender oil is widely recognized for its calming and stress-reducing qualities, while peppermint oil is commonly used to invigorate the senses and relieve headaches. These oils can be inhaled through diffusers, applied topically in diluted forms, or incorporated into massage therapy for a variety of physical and emotional benefits.

The effectiveness of essential oils in aromatherapy is rooted in their ability to interact with the body's systems. When inhaled, the aromatic molecules of essential oils are detected by the olfactory receptors in the nose, sending signals to the brain's limbic system, which governs emotions and memories. This direct connection explains why certain scents can trigger relaxation, enhance mood, or even improve cognitive function. Additionally, when applied to the skin, essential oils can be absorbed into the bloodstream, allowing them to act on specific physical ailments like muscle pain, skin irritation, or respiratory congestion.

One of the defining features of essential oils is their versatility. Different oils are selected depending on the desired outcome, whether it's for physical healing, emotional balance, or mental clarity. For instance, eucalyptus oil is often used to relieve symptoms of colds and flu by clearing nasal passages, while chamomile oil is known for its soothing properties, making it ideal for reducing anxiety or promoting restful sleep. The broad spectrum of essential oils available means that there is an oil for nearly every condition, making aromatherapy a personalized and adaptable approach to wellness.

While essential oils offer numerous benefits, it is important to use them with care. Because of their potency, they should be used in proper dilution, especially when applied topically, to avoid irritation or adverse reactions. It's also essential to choose oils that are of high quality and free from additives or synthetic fragrances to ensure they deliver their full therapeutic potential. Some oils may not be suitable for everyone, such as pregnant women or individuals with certain health conditions, so consulting a healthcare provider is recommended before beginning an aromatherapy regimen.

Essential oils are the heart of aromatherapy because of their ability to connect with both the mind and body in a natural and holistic way. Whether you are seeking relief from physical discomfort, emotional support, or simply a way to enhance your environment, essential oils provide an effective and enjoyable solution. As interest in natural health and wellness continues to grow, these plant-based powerhouses remain at the forefront of alternative healing practices.

Identifying High-Quality Essential Oils

When it comes to aromatherapy, the quality of the essential oils used plays a significant role in their effectiveness and safety. High-quality essential oils are potent, pure, and free from harmful additives or synthetic substances, ensuring that you get the full therapeutic benefits. Identifying top-quality oils requires a keen eye for detail and an understanding of key factors that affect their purity, potency, and overall performance.

One of the most important indicators of quality is the method of extraction. Essential oils are typically obtained through steam distillation or cold pressing, both of which preserve the natural properties of the plant. However, some lower-quality oils may be extracted using chemical solvents, which can leave behind residue that affects both the purity and safety of the oil. Always look for essential oils that specify they are steam-distilled or cold-pressed, as these methods ensure the highest concentration of the plant's beneficial compounds.

Another critical factor to consider is the source of the essential oil. High-quality essential oils are often produced from plants that are grown in their ideal natural environment, where they can thrive without the use of excessive pesticides or chemicals. Organic certification can be an indicator that the plants used to create the oil have been grown without harmful chemicals, further ensuring the purity of the product. If an oil does not come from a reliable source or lacks transparency about its sourcing, it may be worth reconsidering.

The botanical name is another key element in identifying high-quality essential oils. Each essential oil is derived from a specific species of plant, and its botanical name ensures that you are getting the correct oil. For example, lavender oil can come from different species of lavender, and each may have distinct properties. The proper botanical name helps to verify the exact species and guarantee you are using the oil that matches the desired therapeutic effects.

The scent of an essential oil can also reveal much about its quality. Pure essential oils should have a strong, authentic aroma that reflects the natural plant source. If the scent is faint, overly sweet, or synthetic, it could be a sign that the oil has been diluted with a carrier oil or contains artificial fragrances. Additionally, pure essential oils often have subtle variations in scent from batch to batch due to natural differences in the plants used, whereas synthetic oils tend to smell the same each time.

When purchasing essential oils, always check the labeling and transparency of the manufacturer. High-quality brands provide detailed information, such as the country of origin, the distillation process, and the batch number. This level of transparency ensures that the oil has been properly tested and provides insight into its purity and consistency. Reputable brands will also conduct third-party testing, which can confirm the oil's purity, and may even provide a certificate of analysis (COA) upon request.

Price is another factor to consider. While not always an absolute indicator, extremely low-priced oils can often be a red flag. High-quality essential oils require significant resources to produce, and producing them at a low cost may result in the use of subpar ingredients or manufacturing methods. However, high price does not always guarantee quality, so it is essential to look at the other factors listed above in conjunction with the cost.

In summary, identifying high-quality essential oils involves examining the extraction method, sourcing practices, botanical name, scent, labeling transparency, and price. By paying attention to these details, you can ensure that you are investing in pure, effective oils that will provide the best therapeutic benefits for your aromatherapy needs. High-quality essential oils not only support your health and well-being but also enhance your aromatherapy experience with their full potency and natural properties.

Understanding the Different Types of Essential Oils

Essential oils are incredibly diverse, with each type offering unique therapeutic properties that can be used to address a wide range of physical, emotional, and mental well-being needs. These oils are extracted from various parts of plants, such as flowers, leaves, bark, and roots, and are categorized based on their characteristics, uses, and effects. Understanding the different types of essential oils is key to harnessing their full potential in aromatherapy.

One common classification is based on the scent profiles and emotional effects of the oils. **Floral oils** are among the most popular and are known for their sweet, uplifting, and soothing properties. Lavender, one of the most widely used floral essential oils, is renowned for its calming effects, making it ideal for stress relief, anxiety, and sleep support. Rose oil, another floral favorite, is often used for emotional healing, promoting feelings of love, compassion, and relaxation.

Citrus oils are invigorating and refreshing, with a bright, uplifting aroma that can help improve mood and increase energy levels. Oils like lemon, orange, and bergamot are known for their ability to reduce stress, alleviate fatigue, and promote mental clarity. They are often used to boost mood and stimulate the senses, making them perfect for diffusing in the morning or during times of mental fatigue.

Herbal oils have a wide range of uses, often associated with their therapeutic and medicinal qualities. Peppermint oil is one of the most well-known herbal oils, valued for its cooling and soothing effects on headaches, muscle pain, and digestive discomfort. It's also known for its ability to promote mental focus and clarity. Other popular herbal oils include rosemary, which is often used to improve concentration and mental clarity, and basil, which has calming and restorative qualities for the nervous system.

Spicy oils come from plants like cloves, cinnamon, and ginger. These oils tend to have warm, energizing, and stimulating properties, often used to enhance circulation, relieve muscle tension, and support the immune system. Cinnamon essential oil is also known for its antibacterial and antifungal properties, making it a useful oil for cleansing and purifying the air.

Woodsy oils such as sandalwood, cedarwood, and vetiver are often associated with grounding and calming effects. These oils are commonly used in meditation and spiritual practices to help create a sense of balance, stability, and deep relaxation. Sandalwood, in particular, is often included in incense and perfumes for its rich, soothing aroma and is believed to enhance mental clarity and spiritual awareness.

Resin oils are extracted from the sap of trees, such as frankincense and myrrh, and are known for their deep, earthy, and often exotic aromas. These oils have been used for centuries in religious and ceremonial contexts due to their grounding and calming effects. Frankincense, in particular, is valued for its ability to promote relaxation, reduce stress, and support respiratory health.

Finally, **citrus blends and floral blends** are often used in aromatherapy to combine the strengths of multiple oils. Blending oils not only enhances the therapeutic effects of the individual oils but also creates new, complex aromas that can be tailored to specific needs, such as promoting sleep, reducing anxiety, or boosting mood. Many essential oil blends are commercially available, designed for particular outcomes like relaxation, energy, or focus.

Each type of essential oil offers distinct benefits, and knowing how to select the right oil based on your needs can enhance your aromatherapy experience. Whether you are seeking relief from physical discomfort, mental clarity, emotional healing, or simply looking to improve your overall well-being, essential oils provide a natural and effective way to support your health. Their versatility and wide range of applications make them a cornerstone of aromatherapy, offering something for everyone.

Blending Essential Oils

Blending essential oils is an art that allows for the creation of unique and tailored aromatic experiences that enhance the therapeutic benefits of each oil. When oils are blended together, they can complement or amplify each other's properties, producing a more balanced and effective result. The process of blending is not only about crafting pleasing aromas but also about understanding how different oils interact with one another to produce specific effects on the body and mind.

The key to successful blending lies in understanding the different scent families and their corresponding therapeutic properties. Each essential oil can be classified into categories such as floral, citrus, spicy, woodsy, or herbal, and each category brings its own unique qualities to a blend. For example, floral oils like lavender are calming and soothing, while citrus oils like lemon are invigorating and uplifting. By combining oils from complementary scent families, you can create blends that provide a well-rounded therapeutic effect.

When blending essential oils, it's important to consider the **notes** of each oil. Essential oils are generally categorized into top, middle, and base notes, based on how quickly their scent fades once applied. Top notes are the most volatile and tend to evaporate quickly; they are often bright and refreshing, such as citrus or peppermint oils. Middle notes, or heart notes, are the oils that provide the body of the scent and tend to last longer, such as lavender or rosemary. Base notes are the deep, grounding oils that provide richness and longevity to a blend, such as sandalwood or patchouli. A well-balanced blend will incorporate oils from each of these categories to create a harmonious and lasting aroma.

Therapeutic effects are another crucial consideration when creating blends. Essential oils have distinct healing properties that can be combined to target specific health issues. For instance, a blend designed for stress relief might combine the calming effects of lavender (a middle note) with the grounding effects of sandalwood (a base note) and the refreshing qualities of bergamot (a top note). Similarly, a blend to improve focus might pair stimulating oils like peppermint (top note) with clarity-enhancing rosemary (middle note) and grounding vetiver (base note).

Dilution is an essential aspect of blending essential oils, especially for topical use. Essential oils are highly concentrated and can cause irritation if applied directly to the skin without being diluted. A general guideline for dilution is to mix 1-2 drops of essential oil with 1 teaspoon of carrier oil, such as jojoba, coconut, or almond oil. This ensures that the essential oils are safely absorbed into the skin while maintaining their therapeutic effectiveness.

Another important aspect of blending is **personal preference**. Aromatherapy is highly individual, and the scents that work best for one person might not appeal to another. It's essential to experiment with different combinations and adjust ratios to create a blend that resonates with you. You can begin by combining two or three oils and gradually increase the number or adjust the proportions until you find a blend that meets your desired effect.

Blending essential oils can be done in various forms, including creating your own personal perfume, making soothing bath oils, or formulating massage oils. A diffuser is another popular way to enjoy essential oil blends, dispersing the aromas throughout a room and providing therapeutic benefits through inhalation.

In summary, blending essential oils is a creative and practical way to enhance the therapeutic effects of aromatherapy. By understanding the different notes, properties, and potential effects of oils, you can create personalized blends that promote relaxation, boost energy, improve focus, or support your overall well-being. Whether for personal use or in a professional setting, blending offers a way to tailor aromatherapy to meet specific needs and preferences.

The Science Behind Aromatherapy

Aromatherapy is not just a practice of pleasant scents; it is grounded in science, particularly in how the body's senses, brain, and biochemistry interact with the compounds found in essential oils. When essential oils are inhaled or absorbed through the skin, their chemical components have a direct impact on the nervous system, immune system, and other physiological processes, which is why aromatherapy can influence both emotional and physical health.

The primary mechanism of aromatherapy lies in the **olfactory system**. When essential oils are inhaled, the aromatic molecules travel through the nose and bind to receptors in the olfactory bulb, a part of the brain that is closely connected to the **limbic system**. The limbic system is involved in regulating emotions, memories, and certain physiological functions like heart rate, blood pressure, and breathing. This direct connection helps explain why certain scents, such as lavender or peppermint, can have such a powerful impact on mood, stress levels, and emotional states.

Essential oils also influence the **autonomic nervous system**, which controls involuntary bodily functions like heart rate and digestion. For example, inhaling calming oils like lavender and chamomile can activate the parasympathetic nervous system, helping to induce a state of relaxation and reduce the effects of stress and anxiety. On the other hand, stimulating oils like peppermint or citrus can activate the sympathetic nervous system, increasing alertness and energy.

Beyond the olfactory system, essential oils can also be absorbed into the body through the skin. The skin is a permeable barrier, and when essential oils are applied topically (in diluted forms), their chemical constituents can be absorbed and enter the bloodstream. From there, these compounds can influence various systems in the body. For example, **menthol** in peppermint oil has been shown to have cooling and pain-relieving effects when applied to the skin, while **citrus oils** like lemon can act as natural antioxidants, supporting detoxification.

Many essential oils contain bioactive compounds that have been studied for their **antibacterial, antifungal, antiviral, and anti-inflammatory** properties. Tea tree oil, for instance, is widely known for its ability to fight infections and promote skin healing due to its antiseptic properties. Similarly, oils like eucalyptus and thyme are used in respiratory treatments because they have compounds that can help clear the airways and promote deeper breathing.

The **chemical composition** of each essential oil is a major factor in its therapeutic effects. For example, lavender contains a compound called **linalool**, which has been shown in research to have anxiolytic (anxiety-reducing) effects. Similarly, the **limonene** found in citrus oils has been studied for its mood-enhancing and stress-relieving effects. Understanding the specific compounds in each oil allows practitioners to select the most appropriate oils for various health issues.

Research into aromatherapy has also explored its potential for **pain relief** and **wound healing**. Studies have shown that oils like ginger and frankincense can reduce inflammation and may help in managing chronic pain conditions like arthritis. Furthermore, the use of essential oils in wound care has gained interest due to their antimicrobial and healing properties.

While the science behind aromatherapy is still evolving, there is a growing body of evidence supporting its effectiveness as a complementary therapy for a variety of health concerns. The research highlights not only the chemical effects of essential oils but also their ability to influence emotional well-being by interacting with the brain and nervous system.

In summary, aromatherapy is rooted in a fascinating blend of biology and chemistry. The interaction between the body's sensory systems, the limbic system, and the biochemical compounds found in essential oils provides the foundation for its therapeutic benefits. Whether used for physical relief, emotional healing, or mental clarity, the science behind aromatherapy offers a deeper understanding of how these plant-based oils can positively impact health and well-being.

How Aromatherapy Affects the Brain

Aromatherapy has a profound effect on the brain, influencing emotions, mental clarity, and even physical states. This impact is primarily driven by the **olfactory system**, the body's sense of smell, which is directly connected to the **limbic system** in the brain. The limbic system is the emotional center of the brain, responsible for regulating emotions, memories, and behaviors, making it highly receptive to the scents of essential oils.

When aromatic molecules from essential oils are inhaled, they pass through the nasal passages and bind to receptors in the olfactory bulb, a structure located at the top of the nasal cavity. From there, signals are sent to the limbic system, specifically areas like the **amygdala** (which controls emotions) and the **hippocampus** (involved in memory). This direct pathway allows scents to instantly influence mood, evoke memories, and even trigger specific emotional responses.

For example, **lavender** oil, known for its calming and sedative properties, can activate areas of the brain involved in relaxation, leading to a reduction in anxiety and stress. The calming effect of lavender is thought to be linked to the compound **linalool**, which has been shown in studies to reduce levels of cortisol, the hormone associated with stress. Similarly, the fresh, invigorating scent of **peppermint** oil can stimulate the brain, increase alertness, and improve concentration, likely due to its ability to activate the sympathetic nervous system, which controls the body's "fight or flight" response.

Essential oils can also influence **neurotransmitters**, the chemicals that transmit signals in the brain. For example, the scent of **citrus oils** such as lemon and orange has been shown to increase the levels of **serotonin** and **dopamine**, two neurotransmitters involved in mood regulation and feelings of happiness. This is why citrus scents are often used to promote a positive, energized feeling or to uplift mood during times of stress or fatigue.

The effects of aromatherapy are not limited to the limbic system alone. Inhaling essential oils can also affect other parts of the brain, such as the **prefrontal cortex**, which is involved in decision-making and higher cognitive functions. Studies have found that oils like **rosemary** and **sage** can improve cognitive function, memory, and focus by enhancing blood flow to the brain, thus improving mental clarity.

Interestingly, the brain's response to scent is often linked to **emotional memory**, which explains why certain scents can evoke strong, nostalgic memories. For example, the smell of a specific flower or spice may bring back memories of a particular place or time, triggering an emotional response. This is because the olfactory system is one of the few senses that has a direct link to the hippocampus, the brain's memory center. As a result, certain aromas can induce feelings of comfort, happiness, or even relaxation simply by recalling past experiences associated with the scent.

Aromatherapy also interacts with the **autonomic nervous system**, which controls involuntary bodily functions like heart rate, blood pressure, and digestion. By inhaling certain oils, the brain can trigger a relaxation response that calms the nervous system. For example, **frankincense** and **chamomile** oils are known to activate the parasympathetic nervous system, leading to a reduction in heart rate and blood pressure, and promoting a state of deep relaxation.

In summary, the impact of aromatherapy on the brain is a result of complex interactions between scent, the limbic system, neurotransmitters, and other areas of the brain. The therapeutic effects of essential oils are not just about the physical properties of the plants but about their ability to influence brain activity, emotions, and cognitive functions. By using aromatherapy to engage the brain's emotional and sensory centers, individuals can harness the power of essential oils to promote relaxation, improve mood, increase focus, and even enhance memory.

Physical Effects of Aromatherapy

Aromatherapy offers more than just emotional and mental benefits; it also has a significant impact on physical health. The therapeutic properties of essential oils can help alleviate a wide range of physical conditions, from muscle pain and respiratory issues to improving sleep and boosting the immune system. These effects are achieved through the absorption of essential oils into the body either by inhalation or topical application, where their active compounds interact with the body's systems.

One of the most well-known physical effects of aromatherapy is its ability to **relieve pain** and reduce inflammation. Essential oils such as **peppermint, eucalyptus,** and **ginger** are commonly used to ease muscle aches, headaches, and joint pain. **Peppermint oil**, in particular, contains **menthol**, which has a cooling effect on the skin and can help to reduce pain and swelling. When massaged into the affected area, peppermint oil also stimulates blood flow, which can help with muscle recovery after physical exertion.

Aromatherapy also plays a role in **respiratory health**. Oils like **eucalyptus** and **tea tree oil** are often used to clear nasal passages, reduce congestion, and support the respiratory system. **Eucalyptus oil**, for instance, has natural decongestant properties due to its main compound, **1,8-cineole**, which helps to open up airways and facilitate easier breathing. This makes eucalyptus oil a common remedy for colds, flu, and sinus infections. Similarly, **peppermint oil** helps open the airways and can assist in reducing symptoms of asthma or bronchitis.

The **immune system** also benefits from essential oils, as many have natural antibacterial, antiviral, and antifungal properties. **Tea tree oil**, for example, is known for its powerful antimicrobial effects and is often used to prevent and treat infections, both externally on the skin and internally through its antimicrobial properties when inhaled. Oils like **oregano, lemon,** and **frankincense** are also used for their immune-boosting properties, helping to strengthen the body's defenses against illness and promote faster recovery.

Digestive health can be supported through the use of essential oils as well. Oils like **ginger** and **peppermint** are frequently used to help with nausea, indigestion, and bloating. **Peppermint oil**, when used in small amounts, can ease symptoms of irritable bowel syndrome (IBS) and promote smoother digestion. **Ginger oil** is often used to reduce nausea, whether due to motion sickness, morning sickness during pregnancy, or other digestive disturbances.

Essential oils can also have a **detoxifying effect** on the body. Some oils, like **lemon**, **grapefruit**, and **juniper berry**, are known to support the body's natural detoxification processes by stimulating the liver and kidneys, helping to flush out toxins. These oils are often included in blends designed for cleansing or to promote healthy circulation and fluid balance in the body.

Aromatherapy can also help improve **skin health**. Many essential oils are used in skincare for their antiseptic, anti-inflammatory, and healing properties. **Tea tree oil** is a popular treatment for acne due to its antibacterial properties, while **lavender oil** is often applied to soothe minor burns, cuts, and irritations. Oils like **rose** and **frankincense** are known for their anti-aging properties, helping to improve skin elasticity and reduce the appearance of fine lines and wrinkles.

Finally, **improved sleep** is a significant physical benefit that many people seek from aromatherapy. Essential oils such as **lavender, chamomile**, and **cedarwood** have sedative properties that can help calm the nervous system and promote restful sleep. Lavender oil, in particular, has been extensively researched for its ability to improve sleep quality, reduce insomnia, and enhance relaxation before bedtime.

In conclusion, the physical effects of aromatherapy are wide-ranging, from alleviating pain and respiratory issues to boosting immunity and improving skin health. Essential oils work by interacting with the body's sensory systems and biochemical pathways, offering natural and holistic support for various health concerns. By harnessing the power of aromatherapy, individuals can experience relief from common physical ailments and promote overall well-being in a safe and natural way.

Safety Precautions and Guidelines

Aromatherapy can be a highly effective and enjoyable method of supporting physical and emotional well-being, but it's important to follow certain safety precautions and guidelines to ensure the safe and effective use of essential oils. Because essential oils are concentrated extracts from plants, they carry potent bioactive compounds that can have strong effects on the body. Using them improperly can lead to skin irritation, allergic reactions, or even more serious health issues. Here are some essential safety tips to keep in mind when using aromatherapy.

Dilution is Key
Essential oils should never be applied directly to the skin without dilution. They are highly concentrated and can cause skin irritation, redness, or even burns if used undiluted. When applying essential oils topically, always dilute them with a carrier oil such as coconut oil, jojoba oil, or sweet almond oil. A general guideline is to use 1-2 drops of essential oil for every teaspoon of carrier oil for safe topical use. For sensitive areas like the face or delicate skin, a more diluted solution is recommended.

Patch Test First
Before using any essential oil topically, it's crucial to perform a patch test. Apply a small amount of the diluted oil to a discreet area of your skin (such as the inside of your elbow or wrist) and wait for 24 hours to check for any signs of irritation or allergic reaction. If redness, itching, or swelling occurs, avoid using that oil.

Know Your Oils
Not all essential oils are safe for every individual, and some may interact negatively with certain medications or health conditions. Pregnant women, breastfeeding mothers, infants, and people with certain health conditions, such as asthma or epilepsy, should exercise extra caution. Some oils, like **rosemary** or **clary sage**, are not recommended during pregnancy, while others, such as **peppermint**, should be avoided for infants or young children. Always research the specific oils you plan to use and consult with a healthcare professional if you have concerns about potential risks.

Proper Inhalation
While inhalation is a common and effective method for experiencing the benefits of essential oils, it should be done carefully. If using a diffuser, follow the manufacturer's instructions regarding the amount of essential oil to use. Excessive exposure to essential oils in the air can lead to headaches, dizziness, or respiratory irritation, particularly for

individuals with asthma or other respiratory conditions. If you're using an essential oil in a steam inhalation or through direct inhalation from a bottle, it's important to use only a few drops and avoid prolonged exposure.

Storage and Shelf Life

Essential oils are best stored in dark glass bottles to protect them from light and heat, both of which can degrade their potency. Keep them in a cool, dry place, away from direct sunlight, and ensure that the bottles are tightly sealed. Most essential oils have a shelf life of 1-3 years, but citrus oils, such as lemon or orange, tend to have a shorter shelf life and may oxidize faster. Always check for any changes in color, aroma, or consistency, as these can be signs that an oil has gone rancid.

Avoiding Toxic Oils

Some essential oils can be toxic if ingested, applied improperly, or used in excess. For instance, oils like **wintergreen** and **tea tree** can be toxic when swallowed and should never be ingested unless under the guidance of a qualified healthcare provider. **Camphor** and **birch** oils are also highly toxic if consumed. Always keep essential oils out of reach of children, and never ingest essential oils unless directed to do so by a trained professional.

Consult a Professional

If you are new to aromatherapy or have specific health concerns, it's advisable to seek guidance from a qualified aromatherapist or healthcare provider. They can help you select oils that are safe and appropriate for your needs and guide you on how to use them properly. This is especially important if you are using aromatherapy to address specific health conditions, such as chronic pain, respiratory issues, or mental health concerns.

Quality Matters

The quality of essential oils is essential for safety. Always choose oils from reputable suppliers that provide information about the sourcing, distillation process, and purity of the oils. Pure, high-quality essential oils are free from synthetic additives, fillers, and contaminants. Oils labeled as "fragrance oils" or "aromatherapy oils" may contain synthetic ingredients that can cause allergic reactions or offer no therapeutic value.

In summary, aromatherapy can be a wonderful tool for enhancing well-being when used responsibly. By following proper dilution guidelines, conducting patch tests, using high-quality oils, and being aware of any health risks, you can enjoy the many benefits of essential oils safely. When in doubt, always consult a professional to ensure that your use of essential oils is both safe and effective.

Using Essential Oils Safely

Essential oils are powerful plant extracts with a range of therapeutic benefits, but to maximize their effects and minimize risks, it's important to use them safely. These highly concentrated oils can support physical and emotional well-being, but improper use can lead to skin irritation, allergic reactions, or other health issues. Here are key guidelines to ensure that you are using essential oils safely and effectively.

Dilution is Crucial
One of the most important rules when using essential oils is proper dilution. Essential oils are potent and should never be applied directly to the skin without being diluted in a carrier oil like coconut, jojoba, or almond oil. Carrier oils not only help spread the essential oil evenly over the skin but also reduce the risk of irritation or sensitization. A general guideline for dilution is 1-2 drops of essential oil per teaspoon of carrier oil, but this can vary depending on the oil and the intended use.

Always Perform a Patch Test
Before applying any essential oil to a larger area of the skin, it's essential to conduct a patch test to check for any allergic reactions or sensitivity. Apply a small amount of the diluted oil to an inconspicuous part of your body, such as the inside of your elbow or wrist, and wait 24 hours to see if any irritation develops. If you experience redness, itching, or swelling, wash the area with mild soap and water, and avoid using that oil.

Know the Risks for Specific Populations
Certain groups of people, such as pregnant women, infants, young children, and those with specific medical conditions, may need to avoid certain essential oils. Some oils, like **clary sage** and **rosemary**, should be avoided during pregnancy due to their potential to stimulate uterine contractions. Similarly, essential oils like **peppermint** should not be used with infants under 2 years old, as they can be too strong for young children's sensitive skin and respiratory systems. Always consult with a healthcare provider if you are pregnant, nursing, or have underlying health conditions before using essential oils.

Use Essential Oils in Moderation
While essential oils can be highly effective, more is not always better. Overusing essential oils, especially in high concentrations, can cause irritation or other adverse effects. For instance, prolonged exposure to certain oils can cause skin sensitization, which makes the skin more likely to react to subsequent exposure. It's recommended to use essential oils in moderation and follow the guidelines for safe application. If using

them in a diffuser, follow the manufacturer's recommendations on how many drops to use, and avoid running the diffuser for extended periods without breaks.

Inhalation Safety
Inhaling essential oils through a diffuser is a popular and effective way to experience their benefits. However, it's important to ensure proper ventilation and avoid overexposure. Essential oils are potent and can become overwhelming if used in excess. Start with a few drops of essential oil in your diffuser, and use it for no longer than 30 to 60 minutes at a time. People with respiratory issues, such as asthma, should be cautious and choose oils known for their gentler properties, like **lavender** or **chamomile**, and avoid oils with a strong or harsh scent, like **peppermint** or **eucalyptus**, unless recommended by a professional.

Quality Matters
The safety of your aromatherapy experience is directly related to the quality of the essential oils you use. Always choose oils from reputable suppliers who provide information about their sourcing, distillation process, and purity. High-quality oils should be free from synthetic additives, fillers, or contaminants. Look for oils that are labeled as 100% pure, and, if possible, choose organic oils to avoid exposure to pesticides or other harmful chemicals. Avoid products labeled as "fragrance oils," as these often contain synthetic ingredients that do not offer the same therapeutic benefits as pure essential oils.

Storage and Expiration
Proper storage is essential for maintaining the integrity of essential oils. Keep essential oils in dark glass bottles to protect them from light, which can degrade their potency. Store them in a cool, dry place and make sure the bottles are tightly sealed to prevent oxidation. Essential oils typically have a shelf life of 1-3 years, but citrus oils tend to have a shorter shelf life. Be sure to check the oils periodically for changes in scent or appearance, as these may be signs that the oil has gone rancid.

Ingestion and Internal Use
Ingestion of essential oils should be approached with caution and only under the supervision of a trained professional, such as a certified aromatherapist or healthcare provider. Many essential oils can be toxic if swallowed, and the concentration of active compounds can be harmful to the digestive system, liver, or kidneys. Oils like **wintergreen**, **camphor**, and **eucalyptus** are particularly dangerous if ingested. Always use essential oils as directed and avoid self-administering them internally unless under professional guidance.

Avoiding Harmful Reactions
Essential oils should be kept out of the reach of children and pets, as they can be toxic if ingested or improperly applied. Certain oils, such as **tea tree** and **lavender**, can cause severe reactions in animals if they come into contact with them. Always ensure that

essential oils are safely stored, and educate yourself on the potential risks to avoid accidents.

In summary, using essential oils safely is essential to ensuring a positive and therapeutic aromatherapy experience. By following proper dilution guidelines, performing patch tests, understanding the risks for specific groups, using oils in moderation, and choosing high-quality products, you can enjoy the many benefits of essential oils while minimizing the risk of adverse effects. Aromatherapy can be a powerful tool for enhancing well-being when used responsibly and thoughtfully.

Potential Risks and How to Avoid Them

While aromatherapy offers a variety of therapeutic benefits, it's important to recognize that there are potential risks associated with the use of essential oils. These risks are typically linked to misuse, allergies, or interactions with existing health conditions. However, by understanding these risks and following proper safety guidelines, you can enjoy the positive effects of essential oils while minimizing harm.

Skin Irritation and Sensitization
One of the most common risks of using essential oils is skin irritation. Since essential oils are highly concentrated, applying them undiluted to the skin can cause redness, burning sensations, rashes, or blisters. Even oils that are generally considered safe can cause irritation in some individuals, particularly those with sensitive skin. To avoid this risk, always dilute essential oils in a carrier oil, such as jojoba, coconut, or almond oil, before topical application. A general guideline is to use 1-2 drops of essential oil for every teaspoon of carrier oil, but sensitive skin may require a more diluted mixture. Always conduct a patch test on a small area of skin before using any essential oil more widely.

Allergic Reactions
Although rare, some individuals may experience an allergic reaction to certain essential oils. Symptoms can include swelling, itching, hives, or difficulty breathing. Common allergens in essential oils include **citral** (found in citrus oils) and **linalool** (found in lavender and mint oils). To avoid allergic reactions, it is essential to research the specific oils you plan to use and consult with a healthcare provider if you have a history of allergies or asthma. Performing a patch test before full use is also an important preventive measure.

Respiratory Issues
Inhalation of essential oils can sometimes lead to respiratory issues, especially in individuals with asthma, allergies, or other pre-existing lung conditions. Some oils, like **peppermint, eucalyptus**, and **camphor**, contain strong compounds that can irritate the airways, leading to coughing, wheezing, or difficulty breathing. People with asthma or other respiratory conditions should exercise caution and avoid inhaling these oils, or use them in very low concentrations. Always ensure proper ventilation when using essential

oils in a diffuser and consider choosing gentler oils like **lavender** or **chamomile** for those with respiratory sensitivity.

Toxicity from Ingestion

While certain essential oils are widely used in aromatherapy, many are not safe for internal use unless specifically advised by a trained healthcare professional. Ingesting essential oils can be toxic, as their concentrated compounds can irritate the gastrointestinal system or even cause liver and kidney damage. Oils such as **wintergreen**, **camphor**, **oregano**, and **birch** can be particularly dangerous if swallowed. Ingesting essential oils without proper guidance can lead to poisoning, so always consult a professional before using any oils internally. If you suspect accidental ingestion, seek immediate medical attention.

Photosensitivity

Certain essential oils, particularly citrus oils like **bergamot**, **lemon**, and **lime**, can increase sensitivity to sunlight and lead to skin reactions like burns or rashes when exposed to UV rays. This is known as photosensitivity. To avoid this, do not apply these oils to the skin before sun exposure, and always wash off any oils before going outdoors. If you are using these oils, be mindful of your sun exposure and consider applying them in the evening or before bed.

Interactions with Medications

Essential oils can sometimes interact with prescription medications, either reducing their effectiveness or causing adverse effects. For example, oils like **lavender** and **chamomile** may have sedative properties that could interfere with medications for anxiety, depression, or sleep disorders. Additionally, oils like **eucalyptus** and **oregano** may interact with blood-thinning medications, increasing the risk of bleeding. Always consult with your healthcare provider before using essential oils if you are on any long-term medications, especially if you have a chronic health condition.

Essential Oils and Pregnancy

Pregnant women should exercise caution when using essential oils, as some oils can stimulate contractions or cause other complications. Oils like **rosemary**, **clary sage**, and **jasmine** are generally not recommended during pregnancy, particularly in the first trimester. Conversely, oils like **lavender** and **chamomile** are considered safer, but should still be used with caution and under the guidance of a healthcare provider. It's essential to consult with a medical professional before using essential oils during pregnancy to ensure safety for both mother and baby.

Child and Pet Safety

Certain essential oils are not safe for use with children, particularly infants and toddlers. Oils like **peppermint**, **eucalyptus**, and **rosemary** are too potent for young children and can cause respiratory distress or skin irritation. When using essential oils around children, always choose oils that are safe for their age group, such as **lavender** or **chamomile**, and dilute the oils more than you would for adults. Additionally, some essential oils are toxic to pets, especially cats and dogs. **Tea tree oil**, **citrus oils**, and **pine oils** are particularly harmful to animals. Always ensure that essential oils are stored securely and are kept out of reach of pets.

In conclusion, while aromatherapy offers numerous benefits, it's essential to take precautions to minimize risks. By properly diluting essential oils, performing patch tests, avoiding ingestion, and being mindful of potential interactions with medications or health conditions, you can safely enjoy the therapeutic effects of essential oils. Always research and consult with a healthcare provider when needed, especially if you are pregnant, nursing, or dealing with pre-existing health concerns. With the right precautions, you can experience the many physical and emotional benefits of aromatherapy safely and effectively.

Using Aromatherapy for Stress Management

Aromatherapy has become a popular tool for managing stress and promoting relaxation due to its ability to influence both the body and mind. The therapeutic effects of essential oils work by interacting with the **olfactory system**, which sends signals directly to the **limbic system** in the brain—an area responsible for regulating emotions and stress responses. This connection is what makes aromatherapy such an effective and natural method for managing stress.

Several essential oils are known for their calming and stress-relieving properties. **Lavender oil** is one of the most widely used and well-researched oils for stress reduction. Known for its ability to reduce anxiety and promote relaxation, lavender has been shown in studies to lower cortisol levels (the body's primary stress hormone) and induce a sense of calm. Using lavender oil in a diffuser, in a warm bath, or through direct inhalation can help create a peaceful environment that promotes relaxation and reduces the mental and physical symptoms of stress.

Chamomile and **ylang-ylang** are also excellent oils for stress management. Chamomile is widely recognized for its soothing properties and can help calm the nervous system. Its gentle aroma has a sedative effect, making it ideal for easing feelings of tension and anxiety. **Ylang-ylang**, often used in aromatherapy to lift mood and alleviate stress, has been shown to reduce heart rate and blood pressure, which are often elevated during periods of stress.

Bergamot, a citrus oil, is another powerful oil for reducing stress. Unlike many other citrus oils, which tend to be more energizing, bergamot has a calming effect that can improve mood and reduce anxiety. It is often used in blends designed to reduce stress and alleviate symptoms of depression. The combination of its uplifting citrus scent with its calming properties makes it a popular choice for promoting mental clarity and emotional balance.

In addition to these individual oils, **frankincense** is frequently used in meditation and relaxation practices. Known for its grounding properties, frankincense helps quiet the mind and reduce feelings of overwhelm. It has been shown to lower heart rate and blood pressure, both of which can be elevated during times of stress, and it encourages a deeper state of relaxation. **Sandalwood**, another grounding oil, is also used to support meditation and promote a calm, balanced state of mind.

Inhalation is one of the most effective ways to use essential oils for stress management. A diffuser is a great tool for dispersing essential oils into the air, creating a calming environment that promotes relaxation and stress relief. If you don't have a diffuser, simply adding a few drops of essential oil to a cotton ball or inhaling the oil directly from the bottle can provide immediate benefits.

Topical application is another effective method, especially when combined with massage. **Coconut oil** or **jojoba oil** can be used as a carrier oil to dilute essential oils before applying them to the skin. For instance, a blend of lavender, chamomile, and sandalwood diluted in a carrier oil can be massaged into the neck, shoulders, and wrists to alleviate muscle tension and promote a sense of calm. Applying essential oils to pressure points, such as the temples or the base of the neck, can also help soothe the nervous system and reduce stress.

Breathing exercises and **mindfulness practices** can be enhanced with the use of aromatherapy. For example, practicing deep breathing with a few drops of **peppermint** or **eucalyptus** can help clear the mind, reduce stress, and improve focus. These oils are especially useful when feeling mentally fatigued or overwhelmed.

For those who experience **sleep disturbances** due to stress, aromatherapy can help improve sleep quality by promoting relaxation before bed. Essential oils like **lavender**, **cedarwood**, and **vetiver** are known for their ability to calm the mind and prepare the body for restful sleep. Adding a few drops of these oils to a pillow, using them in a diffuser, or applying them topically to the chest and wrists can help create a soothing environment conducive to deep, uninterrupted sleep.

In conclusion, aromatherapy offers a variety of ways to manage stress by leveraging the therapeutic properties of essential oils. Whether through inhalation, topical application, or using oils in combination with other relaxation practices, essential oils can help reduce the physical and emotional symptoms of stress, promote relaxation, and improve overall well-being. By incorporating aromatherapy into your daily routine, you can create a calming environment that supports both mental clarity and emotional balance, helping you navigate the challenges of stress with greater ease.

Understanding How Stress Affects the Body

Stress is a natural response to challenges or threats, but when it becomes chronic, it can have profound effects on both the body and mind. The body's stress response is managed by the **sympathetic nervous system**, which triggers the "fight or flight" response, preparing the body to respond to perceived danger. While this response is beneficial in short bursts, prolonged stress can have a variety of negative consequences on physical health.

When the body is under stress, the **adrenal glands** release hormones like **adrenaline** and **cortisol**. Adrenaline increases heart rate, elevates blood pressure, and boosts energy levels, helping the body react quickly to stressors. Meanwhile, cortisol, often referred to as the "stress hormone," is responsible for regulating a wide range of processes in the body, including metabolism and immune function. Although cortisol is helpful in the short term, chronic elevation can lead to a host of issues, including **immune suppression**, **digestive problems**, and **weight gain**.

Heart and Circulatory System
One of the most immediate physical effects of stress is on the heart. Stress causes the heart rate to increase and blood pressure to rise, as the body prepares to deal with the perceived threat. If this response is prolonged, it can increase the risk of cardiovascular problems, including **hypertension** (high blood pressure), **heart disease**, and **stroke**. Over time, the constant strain on the heart can weaken blood vessels, contributing to the development of heart-related conditions.

Respiratory System
Stress can also have a significant impact on the respiratory system. During stressful situations, the body's breathing rate increases, which can cause shortness of breath or hyperventilation. For individuals with pre-existing respiratory conditions like **asthma** or **chronic obstructive pulmonary disease (COPD)**, stress can exacerbate symptoms and trigger asthma attacks or difficulty breathing. The shallow, rapid breathing that accompanies stress can also lead to a reduction in oxygen intake, which may increase feelings of anxiety and physical discomfort.

Musculoskeletal System
When under stress, the body's muscles tense in response to the fight-or-flight reaction.

While this can be helpful for short-term physical exertion, chronic muscle tension can lead to **headaches, neck pain, shoulder tightness**, and other musculoskeletal problems. Stress-induced muscle tension, especially in the back and shoulders, is one of the leading causes of chronic pain and discomfort. In some cases, stress can even contribute to conditions like **fibromyalgia**, where widespread muscle pain and fatigue are common.

Digestive System
Stress can have a significant impact on the digestive system, often leading to issues like **indigestion, heartburn, nausea**, and **irritable bowel syndrome (IBS)**. Cortisol, when chronically elevated, can disrupt normal digestive processes by decreasing blood flow to the digestive tract, slowing down digestion, and impairing nutrient absorption. For individuals with pre-existing digestive conditions, stress can exacerbate symptoms and trigger flare-ups. Additionally, stress has been linked to changes in gut microbiota, which can affect overall digestion and gut health.

Endocrine System
The endocrine system, which regulates hormones throughout the body, is deeply influenced by stress. Chronic stress can lead to an imbalance in hormones such as cortisol, **insulin**, and **thyroid hormones**. Elevated cortisol levels, for example, can interfere with the body's ability to regulate blood sugar, leading to insulin resistance and, over time, an increased risk of **type 2 diabetes**. Stress can also affect the thyroid, leading to conditions such as **hypothyroidism** or **hyperthyroidism**, both of which can disrupt energy levels, metabolism, and overall health.

Immune System
In the short term, stress can temporarily enhance immune function by stimulating the production of certain immune cells. However, chronic stress has the opposite effect, suppressing the immune system's ability to fight off illness. Prolonged stress leads to the continuous release of cortisol, which, in high amounts, can impair immune function, making the body more susceptible to infections, viruses, and other illnesses. Additionally, stress has been linked to the development of inflammatory conditions, including **arthritis** and **autoimmune diseases**.

Mental Health
Chronic stress doesn't just affect the body physically—it can take a significant toll on mental health. Prolonged exposure to stress can lead to **anxiety, depression, irritability**, and **mood swings**. Stress affects neurotransmitters in the brain, such as **serotonin** and **dopamine**, which regulate mood and emotions. Over time, these imbalances can contribute to mental health disorders, including **anxiety disorders, depression**, and **sleep disturbances**.

In conclusion, while stress is a natural response, prolonged or chronic stress can have wide-reaching effects on nearly every system in the body. The body's constant state of heightened alertness and hormonal imbalance can lead to physical, emotional, and mental health problems if left unaddressed. Managing stress through lifestyle changes, relaxation techniques, and therapeutic practices like **aromatherapy** can help mitigate its harmful effects and support overall health. Understanding the way stress affects the body is the first step in taking control and reducing its impact on daily life.

Which Essential Oils Are Best for Stress Relief

Essential oils can be powerful allies in managing stress, offering natural, soothing relief to calm the mind and body. When used in aromatherapy, specific essential oils interact with the brain's limbic system, promoting relaxation and reducing the symptoms of stress. Here are some of the most effective essential oils for stress relief, each known for their calming and therapeutic properties.

Lavender is perhaps the most well-known and widely used essential oil for stress relief. It has a calming, soothing effect that helps reduce anxiety and promotes relaxation. Lavender oil is particularly effective for helping with sleep, making it a great choice for those who experience stress-related insomnia. Studies have shown that lavender can lower cortisol levels (the body's primary stress hormone) and reduce heart rate, helping to induce a state of calm. It can be used in a diffuser, added to a warm bath, or applied topically (when diluted with a carrier oil) for maximum benefit.

Bergamot, a citrus oil, is unique because it combines uplifting, invigorating qualities with calming effects. It's often used to reduce feelings of anxiety, depression, and nervous tension. Bergamot works by boosting serotonin and dopamine levels in the brain, improving mood and emotional balance. It is commonly used to relieve stress and improve overall mental clarity. Its refreshing yet calming aroma makes it a popular choice for uplifting both the body and mind, and it's often included in blends aimed at relieving stress and anxiety.

Chamomile is another excellent essential oil for stress relief, known for its calming and anti-inflammatory properties. Roman chamomile, in particular, has been used for centuries to alleviate anxiety and promote relaxation. Chamomile oil is gentle and soothing, making it ideal for reducing nervous tension and calming a racing mind. It can be especially helpful for individuals who experience digestive issues related to stress, such as indigestion or bloating, as it also has digestive soothing properties. Chamomile oil can be used in a diffuser, applied topically, or incorporated into a warm bath.

Frankincense, often used in meditation practices, is known for its grounding and centering effects. It helps to calm the mind and body, reducing feelings of overwhelm and promoting a deep sense of peace. Frankincense has the ability to lower heart rate and blood pressure, which can be elevated during times of stress. It is a great choice for those who need help finding mental clarity and grounding during stressful moments. The deep, resinous aroma of frankincense encourages relaxation and is often used to support mindfulness and meditation practices.

Ylang-Ylang is a sweet, floral oil that is particularly effective in reducing feelings of stress and anxiety. It has a sedative effect on the nervous system and is known to promote feelings of calm and emotional stability. Ylang-ylang oil can help reduce high blood pressure, alleviate feelings of frustration, and improve mood. It's often used in aromatherapy to promote relaxation and emotional well-being, making it a great choice for easing stress and anxiety. Its floral aroma can be used in a diffuser or diluted for topical application.

Rose essential oil, with its luxurious, floral scent, is known for its ability to promote emotional healing and relaxation. It is often used to reduce stress caused by emotional trauma or chronic anxiety. Rose oil has a calming effect on the nervous system and can help reduce feelings of agitation and panic. Additionally, it has antidepressant properties, making it a valuable tool for those dealing with anxiety or depressive symptoms related to stress. Rose oil can be diffused, used in massage oils, or added to bath products for a soothing, restorative experience.

Clary Sage is another essential oil with stress-relieving properties, known for its ability to reduce anxiety and balance emotions. It is particularly beneficial for those who experience hormonal imbalances that contribute to stress, such as during PMS or menopause. Clary sage oil promotes relaxation and can help lower blood pressure and calm the nervous system. It is often used to improve mood and provide emotional stability, making it a useful oil for combating stress and irritability.

Vetiver is a grounding, earthy oil that is often used for its calming and sedative properties. It is particularly helpful for individuals who experience nervous exhaustion or feelings of being overwhelmed. Vetiver oil can help to center the mind and promote emotional balance, reducing the physical and mental effects of stress. Its calming properties make it a great choice for those seeking deep relaxation and a sense of peace, especially during times of intense anxiety.

Incorporating these essential oils into your daily routine can provide much-needed relief from stress and anxiety. Whether through diffusing, topical application (when diluted), or adding them to a bath, each oil offers unique benefits that can help promote relaxation, improve mood, and ease the physical symptoms of stress. By selecting the right essential oils for your needs and preferences, you can create a natural, soothing environment that supports your well-being and helps you manage stress more effectively.

Essential Oils for Health and Wellness

Essential oils have been used for centuries to promote health and wellness, offering a natural, holistic approach to improving both physical and emotional well-being. These highly concentrated plant extracts contain bioactive compounds that can positively affect the body and mind. From boosting immunity to enhancing mood, essential oils provide a versatile and effective tool for enhancing overall health.

One of the most popular uses of essential oils is for **immune system support**. **Tea Tree Oil**, known for its powerful antimicrobial properties, is often used to protect against infections and help the body fight off viruses, bacteria, and fungi. Its ability to cleanse and purify the air makes it an excellent choice for supporting respiratory health, especially during cold and flu seasons. **Eucalyptus Oil** is another strong immune booster known for its ability to clear nasal passages and promote easy breathing. It's frequently used to ease symptoms of colds, flu, and sinus congestion, as it helps reduce inflammation in the respiratory system and opens the airways.

For **mental clarity** and **focus**, essential oils like **peppermint** and **rosemary** can be incredibly effective. **Peppermint Oil** is well-known for its invigorating and stimulating properties, promoting mental alertness and improving concentration. It can also be useful for relieving headaches and migraines. **Rosemary Oil** has similar benefits, boosting memory and cognitive function while providing a refreshing, energizing effect. Studies have shown that inhaling rosemary essential oil can improve short-term memory and support mental performance, making it a go-to for those needing a mental pick-me-up.

When it comes to **stress relief** and **emotional well-being**, **lavender** and **chamomile** are among the top choices. **Lavender Oil** is renowned for its calming properties, helping to reduce anxiety and promote relaxation. It has been shown to lower heart rate and blood pressure, creating a soothing effect on both the body and mind. Lavender is also an excellent choice for improving sleep quality, as it helps to calm the nervous system and ease insomnia. **Chamomile Oil**, with its gentle, soothing aroma, is often used to promote relaxation and emotional healing. It can help alleviate feelings of anxiety, reduce nervous tension, and encourage a peaceful state of mind.

For **pain management**, essential oils can offer effective relief. **Ginger Oil** is a well-known natural remedy for **muscle aches** and **joint pain** due to its anti-inflammatory and analgesic properties. It helps improve circulation and can ease symptoms of **arthritis** or **muscle soreness**. **Peppermint Oil**, with its cooling effect, is another favorite for relieving pain. It can be applied topically to reduce tension headaches, sore muscles, or even **fibromyalgia** pain. Additionally, **wintergreen** and **lavender** oils are commonly used for their soothing and pain-relieving qualities, offering natural alternatives to over-the-counter pain medications.

When it comes to **skin health**, essential oils like **tea tree, frankincense,** and **rose** are excellent choices. **Tea Tree Oil** is widely used for its antibacterial and antifungal properties, making it an effective treatment for acne, eczema, and minor skin infections. **Frankincense Oil** is known for its rejuvenating and anti-aging effects. It helps promote skin cell regeneration, reduce the appearance of scars, and improve the tone and texture of the skin. **Rose Oil**, with its nourishing properties, is commonly used for its anti-inflammatory and skin-soothing effects. It's known to hydrate and restore the skin while reducing redness and irritation.

For **digestive health**, essential oils like **peppermint, ginger,** and **lemon** are particularly helpful. **Peppermint Oil** has been widely studied for its ability to alleviate symptoms of **irritable bowel syndrome (IBS)**, bloating, and indigestion. It works by relaxing the muscles in the digestive tract, allowing for smoother digestion. **Ginger Oil** is another excellent choice for improving digestion and relieving nausea. It's often used to treat motion sickness, morning sickness during pregnancy, and digestive discomfort. **Lemon Oil** is known to stimulate the digestive system and act as a natural detoxifier, supporting the liver and promoting the elimination of toxins.

For **skin detoxification**, essential oils such as **lemongrass, juniper berry,** and **grapefruit** can assist in flushing out toxins from the body and promoting clear skin. **Lemongrass Oil** has detoxifying properties that help reduce the appearance of blemishes and balance oil production in the skin. **Juniper Berry Oil** is often used to support lymphatic drainage and improve circulation, helping to remove waste from the body and prevent skin congestion. **Grapefruit Oil** is a natural diuretic and detoxifier that supports the body's natural cleansing processes while promoting healthy skin.

Essential oils are a versatile and natural way to enhance both physical and emotional health. Whether used for immune support, mental clarity, pain relief, or skin care, these plant-based oils offer a variety of benefits for overall wellness. By incorporating essential oils into your daily routine, you can take a proactive approach to your health, fostering balance, vitality, and well-being. Whether diffused, applied topically, or used in a bath, essential oils can make a meaningful contribution to your health and wellness journey.

Boosting the Immune System With Essential Oils

Essential oils have long been used in aromatherapy to support the body's natural defenses, offering a natural and effective way to boost the immune system. These oils contain potent compounds that have antibacterial, antiviral, antifungal, and anti-inflammatory properties, making them valuable tools in promoting overall health and preventing illness. By using essential oils in various forms, such as inhalation, topical application, or in a diffuser, you can enhance your body's ability to fight off infections and maintain a balanced immune system.

One of the most well-known essential oils for immune support is **Tea Tree Oil**. Revered for its strong antimicrobial properties, tea tree oil is widely used to combat bacterial, viral, and fungal infections. Its ability to purify the air makes it an excellent choice for respiratory support, especially during cold and flu season. Inhaling tea tree oil or diffusing it into the air can help clear nasal passages and prevent the spread of germs. Topically, it can be diluted and applied to wounds, cuts, or blemishes to help prevent infection and promote healing.

Another powerful essential oil for immune support is **Eucalyptus Oil**. Known for its decongestant and antiviral properties, eucalyptus oil is often used to clear the airways, making it particularly beneficial for respiratory health. It helps to reduce inflammation in the respiratory system and can support the body's defense against colds, flu, and other respiratory infections. Eucalyptus oil is commonly used in steam inhalations or diffusers to promote easy breathing and purify the air. When diluted and applied to the chest or throat, it can help relieve symptoms of congestion and cough.

Lemon Oil is a refreshing, citrusy oil known for its detoxifying properties. It has natural antiseptic and antibacterial effects that help cleanse the body and support immune function. Lemon oil can help boost the lymphatic system, promoting the removal of toxins and improving circulation. It also has mood-boosting qualities, which can be helpful for reducing stress—one of the major factors that can weaken the immune system. Lemon oil can be diffused to purify the air and lift your spirits or used in a detoxifying bath to support the body's natural cleansing processes.

Oregano Oil is another essential oil with strong immune-boosting properties. It contains compounds like **carvacrol** and **thymol**, which have been shown to possess antiviral, antibacterial, and antifungal effects. Oregano oil is particularly useful in combating infections and supporting the immune system during illness. Because it is very potent, it should always be diluted with a carrier oil before applying to the skin. Ingesting oregano oil should only be done under the supervision of a healthcare professional due to its strong concentration.

Thyme Oil is a powerful antibacterial and antiviral oil, making it a great choice for strengthening the immune system and preventing infections. It is particularly effective in supporting the respiratory and digestive systems. Thyme oil has been traditionally used to fight off colds and flu, as well as to support digestion and ease stomach discomfort. Diffusing thyme oil or applying it topically (in diluted form) can help reduce symptoms of respiratory infections and strengthen the body's immune response.

Frankincense Oil is not only revered for its spiritual and grounding properties but also for its ability to support immune health. This ancient oil has anti-inflammatory and antimicrobial properties that help the body fight off infections and reduce inflammation. Frankincense can be used to strengthen the immune system by promoting the production of white blood cells, which are essential in fighting off pathogens. It also helps to reduce stress, which is important for maintaining a healthy immune response.

Peppermint Oil is another essential oil that can aid in immune support, particularly by improving circulation and stimulating the immune system. It has cooling and soothing effects, which can help relieve inflammation, headaches, and respiratory issues. Peppermint oil is particularly helpful when used in a diffuser or applied topically to alleviate symptoms of congestion, sore throat, and sinus pressure. Its antibacterial properties also make it useful for protecting the body from germs and bacteria.

In addition to using these individual essential oils, many people find that blending oils together can enhance their immune-boosting effects. A combination of **tea tree**, **eucalyptus**, and **lemon** oils, for example, can be a powerful blend to purify the air, clear the sinuses, and prevent the spread of harmful bacteria and viruses. A blend of **frankincense**, **lemon**, and **peppermint** can also support respiratory health, reduce inflammation, and improve overall immunity.

Essential oils can be used in a variety of ways to boost the immune system. **Diffusing** essential oils is one of the most effective methods, as it allows the oils to be inhaled, where they can act on the respiratory system and strengthen the body's defenses. **Topical application** is another great way to incorporate essential oils into your wellness routine, but always remember to dilute the oils with a carrier oil like coconut or jojoba oil to avoid skin irritation. **Steam inhalation**, by adding a few drops of essential oil to hot water and inhaling the steam, can be particularly useful for respiratory support.

In conclusion, essential oils are a natural and effective way to boost the immune system and protect the body from illness. With their powerful antibacterial, antiviral, antifungal, and anti-inflammatory properties, these oils provide a holistic approach to enhancing the body's ability to fight infections. Whether used in a diffuser, in a bath, or applied topically, essential oils can be a valuable tool in supporting health and wellness, especially during cold and flu season. By integrating these oils into your daily routine, you can help strengthen your immune system and improve your overall vitality.

Essential Oils for Pain Management

Essential oils are a popular and natural option for managing pain, offering a wide range of therapeutic properties that can help alleviate discomfort from conditions such as muscle soreness, joint pain, headaches, and even chronic pain. These potent plant extracts work by interacting with the body's sensory and nervous systems, providing relief through both **anti-inflammatory** and **analgesic** effects. Whether applied topically, inhaled, or used in a bath, essential oils can be a soothing remedy for many types of pain.

One of the most widely used essential oils for pain relief is **Peppermint Oil**. Known for its cooling and soothing properties, peppermint oil contains **menthol**, a compound that helps to relax muscles, ease tension, and relieve headaches. It is particularly effective for **tension headaches** and **migraines** when applied to the temples, forehead, or back of the neck. Peppermint oil also has **analgesic** properties, making it useful for alleviating sore muscles, joint pain, and cramps. When diluted and massaged into affected areas, it can provide quick relief from muscle pain and inflammation.

Lavender Oil is another highly effective oil for pain management, particularly for **muscle aches**, **joint pain**, and **stress-induced tension**. Lavender is well known for its calming and relaxing properties, but it also has **anti-inflammatory** and **analgesic** effects that can help reduce pain and swelling. It is particularly beneficial for easing the discomfort of conditions like **fibromyalgia** and **arthritis**. When used in a warm bath or applied topically to sore muscles, lavender oil can help promote relaxation and relieve both physical and emotional stress, which often contributes to pain.

For **joint pain** and **arthritis**, **Eucalyptus Oil** is often recommended. Its active compound, **1,8-cineole**, has both **anti-inflammatory** and **analgesic** properties, making eucalyptus oil effective for reducing inflammation and relieving pain. It works by increasing blood flow to affected areas, which helps to reduce swelling and promote healing. Eucalyptus oil can be applied topically (after proper dilution) or inhaled through steam to help relieve pain associated with **rheumatoid arthritis, osteoarthritis**, and **muscle stiffness**.

Ginger Oil, derived from the root of the ginger plant, is highly effective for treating **muscle soreness**, **joint pain**, and **inflammation**. Ginger has natural **anti-inflammatory** compounds, such as **gingerol**, which help reduce swelling and discomfort. It is particularly useful for individuals with **osteoarthritis** and **rheumatoid arthritis** due to its ability to relieve stiffness and joint pain. Ginger oil can be diluted with a carrier oil and massaged into the affected areas, providing relief and improving circulation. Additionally, it can help alleviate **nausea** associated with pain, making it a great option for individuals who experience gastrointestinal distress due to chronic pain.

Rosemary Oil is another excellent essential oil for easing **muscle pain** and **arthritis**. Rosemary contains compounds like **camphor** and **borneol**, which have **anti-inflammatory** and **analgesic** effects. Rosemary oil is particularly beneficial for easing tension and reducing pain in the neck, back, and shoulders. It also helps to increase circulation, which can reduce inflammation and promote healing in sore muscles and joints. Diffusing rosemary oil or applying it topically to the affected area can provide significant relief from discomfort and stiffness.

Frankincense Oil is widely recognized for its ability to reduce inflammation and relieve pain associated with **arthritis, muscle spasms,** and **injuries**. Its **anti-inflammatory** properties help to reduce swelling, while its **analgesic** properties provide pain relief. Frankincense oil can be used in aromatherapy to reduce pain, or it can be applied topically (when diluted) to sore muscles, joints, and ligaments. This oil also has a grounding, calming effect, which can help alleviate stress and emotional tension that may exacerbate physical pain.

For those dealing with **headaches** and **migraines**, **Basil Oil** is an excellent option. Basil has natural **analgesic** and **anti-inflammatory** properties that can help reduce the intensity of tension headaches. It works by improving circulation, reducing muscle tightness in the head and neck, and calming the nervous system. Basil oil can be applied to the temples, neck, and shoulders to ease pain or inhaled through steam to help alleviate headache symptoms.

Wintergreen Oil is another effective oil for pain relief, particularly for **muscle pain** and **joint inflammation**. It contains **methyl salicylate**, a compound with properties similar to **aspirin**, which makes it highly effective for reducing pain and inflammation. Wintergreen oil is commonly used in massage blends to relieve sore muscles and improve circulation. It should always be used with caution and diluted properly, as it can be quite strong and may cause irritation if not properly prepared.

Clary Sage Oil is particularly beneficial for **pain management** related to **menstrual cramps** and **muscle spasms**. It helps to relax the muscles, reduce inflammation, and balance hormonal fluctuations that can cause pain. Clary sage oil can be used in a warm bath or massaged into the lower abdomen to ease cramping and discomfort associated with menstruation. It also has a calming effect that can help relieve stress-related tension and muscle tightness.

Incorporating essential oils into your pain management routine can provide natural, effective relief for various types of discomfort. Whether through topical application, inhalation via a diffuser, or use in a warm bath, essential oils offer versatile and therapeutic options for easing pain. Always remember to dilute essential oils with a carrier oil when applying them topically and to conduct a patch test to ensure you don't have any skin sensitivities. By using these oils responsibly, you can experience the natural, healing power of aromatherapy and manage pain in a holistic, gentle way.

Improving Sleep Quality Through Aromatherapy

Aromatherapy has long been recognized as an effective way to promote better sleep, offering natural solutions for those struggling with insomnia or poor sleep quality. Essential oils interact with the brain's limbic system, which governs emotions and sleep regulation, helping to calm the nervous system, reduce anxiety, and promote a sense of relaxation. Using essential oils in a diffuser, on pillows, or through topical application can enhance your sleep environment and make it easier to unwind after a long day.

One of the most well-known essential oils for sleep is **Lavender Oil**. Numerous studies have shown that lavender is effective in improving sleep quality by promoting relaxation and reducing anxiety. The scent of lavender has a calming effect that helps lower heart rate and blood pressure, creating the perfect environment for restful sleep. It is particularly useful for individuals who have trouble falling asleep due to stress or anxiety. Lavender oil can be diffused into the air, added to a pillow, or used in a warm bath before bedtime to encourage deeper, more restorative sleep.

Chamomile Oil is another excellent choice for improving sleep quality, especially for those who experience anxiety or restlessness before bed. Chamomile is well-known for its sedative properties, helping to relax both the mind and body. **Roman chamomile**, in particular, is often used in aromatherapy to calm the nervous system and promote a peaceful night's sleep. Its gentle, floral aroma is soothing, making it a great choice for creating a calming bedtime ritual. You can use chamomile oil in a diffuser or mix it with a carrier oil and apply it to pulse points like the wrists and temples.

Bergamot Oil, derived from the rind of the bergamot orange, is a citrus oil that stands out for its ability to reduce anxiety while also uplifting the spirit. It is one of the few citrus oils with calming properties, making it perfect for bedtime relaxation. Bergamot has been shown to decrease cortisol levels (the body's stress hormone) and promote feelings of calm and emotional balance. It is especially helpful for those who experience **stress-related insomnia**, where racing thoughts and nervous tension keep them from falling asleep. Bergamot can be used in a diffuser, or a few drops can be added to a warm bath for a soothing pre-sleep ritual.

Ylang-Ylang Oil, with its sweet floral aroma, is another excellent choice for promoting relaxation and better sleep. Ylang-ylang has a calming effect on the nervous system and is often used to alleviate feelings of anxiety and stress. It can help reduce heart rate and lower blood pressure, making it easier to unwind before bed. Ylang-ylang oil is especially useful for individuals who experience **emotional unrest** or **mood swings** that interfere with their ability to relax. Diffusing ylang-ylang or using it in a sleep blend can encourage a peaceful transition into sleep.

Sandalwood Oil is known for its grounding and calming effects, making it a great choice for promoting deep sleep. Its rich, earthy aroma can help reduce feelings of restlessness and promote mental clarity, allowing the mind to slow down and relax before sleep. Sandalwood is often used in meditation and mindfulness practices due to its ability to calm the mind and reduce anxiety. Diffusing sandalwood or applying it topically, when diluted with a carrier oil, can help improve the quality of your sleep and enhance relaxation.

Clary Sage Oil is another powerful oil for improving sleep, particularly for those who suffer from **hormonal imbalances** that affect their sleep patterns, such as during menopause or menstruation. Clary sage has a relaxing, sedative effect on the body and mind and can help reduce feelings of stress, tension, and anxiety. It's also known for its ability to promote emotional balance, which can be particularly helpful if **emotional stress** is contributing to poor sleep. Clary sage oil can be used in a diffuser or diluted with a carrier oil and applied to the chest or wrists for relaxation.

In addition to individual oils, **blends** of essential oils can be particularly effective in improving sleep quality. A blend of **lavender**, **chamomile**, and **ylang-ylang** is often used to create a calming environment conducive to sleep. These oils work synergistically to promote relaxation, reduce anxiety, and ease both the mind and body into restful sleep. Similarly, a blend of **bergamot**, **sandalwood**, and **frankincense** can help ground the mind, reduce stress, and promote a deep, peaceful sleep.

Incorporating aromatherapy into your bedtime routine can make a significant difference in the quality of your sleep. Whether you choose to use a diffuser, add essential oils to your pillow or bedding, or use them in a relaxing bath or massage, the benefits of aromatherapy for sleep are far-reaching. Essential oils help create a peaceful, serene environment that encourages relaxation and supports the body's natural sleep cycle. With consistent use, aromatherapy can help improve sleep quality, reduce anxiety, and provide you with the restful, rejuvenating sleep you need to feel your best.

Aromatherapy for Emotional Balancing

Aromatherapy is an effective tool for emotional balancing, helping to stabilize mood, reduce anxiety, and enhance overall emotional well-being. Through the use of essential oils, aromatherapy can stimulate the brain's limbic system, which plays a key role in regulating emotions, memories, and behaviors. The power of scent has a profound impact on the nervous system, helping to calm, uplift, or ground the emotions based on the specific oils used. By incorporating aromatherapy into your daily routine, you can create a more balanced, calm, and positive emotional state.

One of the most widely used oils for emotional balancing is **Lavender Oil**. Known for its calming properties, lavender has been shown to reduce stress and anxiety, promoting relaxation and emotional stability. Its soothing aroma helps to regulate the nervous system, lowering heart rate and blood pressure. Lavender oil is particularly effective for those experiencing **emotional overwhelm** or **irritability**, as it helps to calm the mind and bring a sense of peaceful balance. It can be diffused in the air, applied topically, or added to a warm bath for maximum benefit.

Bergamot Oil, derived from the rind of the citrus fruit, is a powerful oil for boosting mood and balancing emotions. It is often used to relieve **feelings of sadness** and **anxiety** while promoting a sense of optimism and relaxation. Bergamot helps to reduce **cortisol** levels, the body's primary stress hormone, allowing the body to return to a balanced emotional state. It is also known to uplift the spirit, making it particularly useful for those experiencing **depression** or **mood swings**. Bergamot can be used in a diffuser, added to a calming bath, or applied to pulse points to restore emotional balance and reduce feelings of nervous tension.

For **stress management** and **mood enhancement**, **Frankincense Oil** is an excellent choice. Frankincense has grounding and calming effects on the mind, helping to reduce feelings of anxiety, stress, and mental clutter. It has been used for centuries in spiritual practices due to its ability to help deepen meditation and promote emotional healing. Frankincense encourages a sense of inner peace, making it ideal for those seeking emotional clarity and calmness. Whether used in meditation, diffused into the air, or applied to the skin, frankincense can provide emotional support during times of stress.

Ylang-Ylang Oil is a sweet floral oil that works wonders for balancing emotions and enhancing feelings of happiness. It is particularly effective for those experiencing emotional distress due to hormonal imbalances, such as during **PMS** or **menopause**. Ylang-ylang helps to regulate the nervous system, reduce anxiety, and promote feelings of joy. It is also known to be a natural **antidepressant**, making it useful for alleviating feelings of sadness or irritability. The gentle, uplifting aroma of ylang-ylang can be diffused or used in a massage oil to promote emotional balance and restore a sense of calm.

Rose Oil, with its rich, luxurious scent, is another essential oil known for its ability to restore emotional harmony. It is widely used for its **heart-opening** qualities, helping to foster love, compassion, and emotional healing. Rose oil is particularly beneficial for those dealing with **emotional trauma**, **grief**, or **anxiety**, as it works to soothe the emotional body and bring feelings of comfort. The gentle properties of rose oil help to stabilize mood, calm emotional turbulence, and promote a sense of emotional well-being.

For those needing a **grounding** or **centering** effect, **Sandalwood Oil** is a great choice. Its deep, earthy aroma has a calming effect on the mind and emotions, making it ideal for reducing feelings of restlessness or agitation. Sandalwood helps to promote a sense of **inner peace**, emotional stability, and clarity. It can be used to ease anxiety and stress or help those who feel ungrounded or overwhelmed. Sandalwood oil is often used in meditation and spiritual practices to enhance mindfulness and emotional presence.

Clary Sage Oil is especially effective for emotional balancing in individuals experiencing **hormonal fluctuations**. It has a calming, soothing effect on both the mind and body, helping to alleviate mood swings, irritability, and anxiety. Clary sage is known for its ability to balance emotions by calming the nervous system and promoting emotional harmony. It is particularly beneficial for women dealing with **PMS**, **menopausal symptoms**, or **stress-related hormonal imbalances**. Clary sage can be used in a diffuser, bath, or diluted and applied to the skin for emotional support.

Geranium Oil, with its sweet floral aroma, is a wonderful essential oil for promoting emotional stability and mental clarity. Geranium is particularly useful for balancing the **emotional energy** and encouraging emotional healing. It helps to uplift the spirit, reduce feelings of anxiety, and calm mood swings. Geranium oil can also help foster a positive outlook by boosting **self-esteem** and **emotional resilience**, making it a great choice for those dealing with feelings of **low confidence** or **self-doubt**.

By incorporating these essential oils into your daily routine, you can effectively support your emotional well-being. Aromatherapy offers a natural and holistic approach to emotional balancing, helping to ease stress, promote relaxation, and enhance mental clarity. Whether you choose to use these oils through diffusion, topical application, or in a soothing bath, essential oils can provide the emotional support needed to navigate daily challenges with greater ease and resilience.

Essential Oils for Anxiety and Depression

Aromatherapy offers a natural and effective way to manage anxiety and depression, two conditions that can be debilitating for many individuals. The use of essential oils can help alleviate the emotional and physical symptoms associated with these conditions by interacting with the body's sensory systems and influencing the brain's limbic system, which controls emotions and memory. Certain essential oils are particularly known for their ability to reduce stress, promote relaxation, and uplift mood, providing relief from the negative effects of anxiety and depression.

Lavender Oil is one of the most widely used and researched essential oils for managing both anxiety and depression. Known for its calming and sedative properties, lavender helps to relax the nervous system, reduce heart rate, and lower blood pressure. Lavender oil has been shown in numerous studies to be effective in alleviating symptoms of **generalized anxiety** and **depression**, promoting a sense of peace and relaxation. Whether used in a diffuser, added to a warm bath, or applied to the skin (when diluted with a carrier oil), lavender oil can help soothe emotional tension and promote better sleep—something often disrupted by anxiety and depression.

Bergamot Oil, derived from the rind of the citrus fruit, is another powerful essential oil for easing anxiety and improving mood. Unlike many other citrus oils that are more uplifting, bergamot has a unique combination of both **calming** and **mood-enhancing** properties. It is known to reduce **cortisol** levels (the body's stress hormone), helping to relieve tension and emotional distress. Bergamot oil is particularly effective for those dealing with **stress-induced anxiety**, as it can induce relaxation while simultaneously lifting mood and reducing feelings of sadness. Diffusing bergamot or applying it to pulse points can help balance emotions and promote mental clarity.

Frankincense Oil is often used for its grounding properties, making it ideal for calming the mind and alleviating the symptoms of anxiety and depression. Frankincense helps reduce **nervous tension** and **mental fatigue**, making it a great choice for those struggling with persistent worry or feelings of overwhelm. It has the ability to promote a sense of deep calm and emotional stability, which can be especially beneficial for individuals who experience intense anxiety or feelings of sadness. The grounding aroma of frankincense makes it particularly useful for those seeking to find emotional balance in times of emotional distress.

Clary Sage Oil is another essential oil known for its ability to reduce anxiety and elevate mood. It has **mood-stabilizing** effects that can help alleviate symptoms of **depression**, especially when it's related to **hormonal fluctuations**, such as in PMS or menopause. Clary sage helps to calm the nervous system, promote relaxation, and provide emotional support during times of stress. The comforting, herbaceous aroma of clary sage can help uplift the spirit, reduce feelings of irritability, and encourage emotional harmony, making it particularly helpful for individuals dealing with **mood swings** or **emotional volatility** associated with anxiety and depression.

Ylang-Ylang Oil, with its sweet, floral scent, is known for its **antidepressant** and **anxiolytic** effects. It is particularly beneficial for those who experience **low mood** or **nervous tension**. Ylang-ylang helps to lift the spirit, promote relaxation, and reduce feelings of anger and frustration, which are often associated with depression and anxiety. This oil is also known to help balance emotions, calm the mind, and reduce feelings of emotional overload. Ylang-ylang can be used in a diffuser, applied to the skin in a diluted form, or added to a bath to help reduce anxiety and promote a sense of well-being.

Rosemary Oil is another essential oil that can help alleviate the mental fatigue and cognitive fog often experienced during periods of anxiety or depression. Known for its **clarifying** and **stimulating** properties, rosemary helps to improve mental clarity and reduce feelings of **exhaustion**. It also helps to lift mood and reduce feelings of negativity, which can be common in depressive states. By stimulating the circulation of both blood and oxygen in the brain, rosemary oil helps to enhance focus, alleviate mental sluggishness, and promote emotional resilience, making it a helpful oil for individuals who are feeling mentally drained.

Chamomile Oil, especially **Roman chamomile**, is well-known for its **calming** and **sedative** properties. It has a gentle effect on the nervous system and is particularly effective in reducing symptoms of **stress** and **anxiety**. Chamomile oil promotes deep relaxation and can help relieve feelings of frustration, nervousness, and unease. Its ability to soothe both the body and mind makes it an excellent oil for those struggling with sleep disturbances caused by anxiety or depression. Chamomile can be diffused before bedtime or used in a relaxing massage to promote emotional well-being and enhance sleep quality.

Geranium Oil has a balancing effect on both the mind and emotions, making it useful for those dealing with **stress** and **mood imbalances**. Known for its **hormonal-balancing** properties, geranium oil helps to promote emotional stability, reduce irritability, and relieve feelings of sadness or anxiety. It is especially effective in alleviating **emotional exhaustion** and **mood swings**, often providing a sense of emotional support during challenging times. Geranium oil is best used in a diffuser or in a soothing bath to create an environment of emotional balance and comfort.

Using these essential oils in combination or individually can provide natural relief from the emotional and physical symptoms of anxiety and depression. Whether diffused, inhaled, applied to pulse points, or used in a relaxing bath, essential oils offer a non-invasive, effective approach to emotional healing. By incorporating these oils into a daily routine, individuals can support their emotional well-being, reduce stress, and enhance their overall mental health. Always ensure to dilute oils properly for topical use and consult with a healthcare provider before using essential oils if you have underlying health concerns or are pregnant.

Aromatherapy for Emotional Wellbeing

Aromatherapy is a powerful tool for promoting emotional well-being, offering a natural and holistic approach to improving mood, reducing stress, and supporting overall mental health. The essential oils used in aromatherapy interact with the brain's limbic system, which governs emotions, behavior, and memory. This direct connection allows specific scents to have a profound effect on emotional health by influencing the nervous system, reducing anxiety, and boosting feelings of happiness and relaxation.

Lavender Oil is one of the most commonly used essential oils for promoting emotional well-being. Known for its calming properties, lavender helps to soothe the nervous system, reduce anxiety, and improve sleep quality. Studies have shown that inhaling lavender oil can significantly reduce symptoms of **stress** and **depression** by lowering cortisol levels (the body's stress hormone) and promoting a sense of calm. Lavender oil can be used in a diffuser, added to a bath, or applied topically (when diluted) to pulse points for relaxation and emotional balance.

Bergamot Oil is another essential oil that supports emotional health, particularly by reducing feelings of anxiety and improving mood. Unlike other citrus oils that are more invigorating, bergamot offers a balance of uplifting and calming effects. It has been shown to reduce **cortisol** levels and increase the production of **serotonin**, the neurotransmitter responsible for regulating mood and promoting happiness. Bergamot oil is especially helpful for those dealing with **stress-related emotional imbalances** and can be used in aromatherapy to alleviate symptoms of **mild depression** and **anxiety**.

Frankincense Oil, with its rich, grounding aroma, is another excellent choice for emotional wellness. Often used in meditation, frankincense helps to calm the mind, reduce feelings of stress, and promote a deep sense of relaxation. It has been shown to help ease **mental fatigue** and encourage clarity and emotional resilience. By helping to slow the heart rate and reduce blood pressure, frankincense can induce a state of calmness that supports emotional healing. It can be used in a diffuser or applied topically to pulse points to improve emotional well-being and foster a peaceful state of mind.

Ylang-Ylang Oil is a sweet, floral oil known for its ability to uplift the spirit and promote emotional balance. It is often used to help alleviate feelings of **anxiety**, **stress**, and **mood swings**. Ylang-ylang's calming properties help reduce nervous tension while 's mood-boosting effects create a sense of emotional stability and well-being. The sweet floral scent has been shown to help reduce heart rate and promote feelings of relaxation and joy, making it ideal for those dealing with emotional distress. Diffusing ylang-ylang or using it in a massage oil blend can help lift the mood and support emotional health.

Rose Oil, with its luxurious floral aroma, has long been used to promote emotional healing and well-being. Rose oil helps balance emotions, reduce feelings of sadness, and promote feelings of self-love and compassion. It is particularly effective for individuals dealing with **grief, emotional trauma**, or **stress**. Rose oil helps calm the nervous system and encourage emotional healing by promoting a sense of peace and inner harmony. It can be used in aromatherapy to create a calming environment, reduce stress, and foster emotional healing.

Geranium Oil is an excellent essential oil for emotional support, especially when it comes to balancing mood and reducing feelings of anxiety or **stress**. Geranium has been shown to have **anti-anxiety** and **mood-lifting** effects, making it ideal for individuals who experience **emotional instability** or **irritability**. It is often used to boost self-esteem and emotional resilience, helping individuals feel more centered and balanced. Geranium oil can be diffused to create a calm, balanced atmosphere or added to a bath for emotional relaxation and rejuvenation.

Chamomile Oil, particularly **Roman chamomile**, is well-known for its ability to calm the mind and soothe the emotions. It is often used to alleviate **stress** and **anxiety** by helping to relax the nervous system and promote mental clarity. Chamomile oil has a gentle, soothing effect that reduces feelings of **restlessness** and encourages a more peaceful state of mind. It is particularly helpful for those who experience **nervous tension** or **insomnia** due to emotional stress. Chamomile can be diffused in the evening to help with relaxation or used in a bath to support emotional balance and restful sleep.

Clary Sage Oil is another essential oil that is commonly used to promote emotional well-being, particularly for those dealing with **stress** or **hormonal imbalances**. It has a calming, soothing effect on both the mind and body, helping to reduce anxiety and promote emotional stability. Clary sage also helps to alleviate **mood swings** and is often used to support **emotional balance** during times of hormonal changes, such as PMS or menopause. The oil can be used in aromatherapy to reduce emotional tension and enhance overall emotional resilience.

In addition to using individual oils, creating blends of essential oils can enhance their therapeutic effects on emotional well-being. For example, a blend of **lavender, frankincense**, and **ylang-ylang** can help promote relaxation, reduce anxiety, and improve mood. Similarly, a combination of **bergamot, chamomile**, and **geranium** can help balance emotions, relieve stress, and foster emotional healing.

Aromatherapy can be incorporated into your daily routine in several ways. Essential oil can be diffused into the air, creating a calming and uplifting environment. They can also be applied topically (with proper dilution) to pulse points, temples, or the back of the neck for targeted emotional support. Adding essential oils to a warm bath can also help ease emotional tension and promote relaxation. Regular use of essential oils can help improve emotional well-being, reduce anxiety, and promote a positive mindset, making aromatherapy a powerful tool for emotional self-care and balance.

Aromatherapy for Skin Care

Aromatherapy offers a natural and holistic approach to skin care, utilizing essential oils to address a variety of skin concerns. These potent plant extracts contain bioactive compounds that can soothe, heal, and rejuvenate the skin. Whether you're looking to combat acne, reduce the appearance of scars, or enhance skin hydration, essential oils provide effective solutions for maintaining healthy, glowing skin. By incorporating essential oils into your skincare routine, you can nourish your skin while reaping the benefits of aromatherapy's therapeutic properties.

Tea Tree Oil is one of the most popular essential oils for skincare, particularly for treating **acne** and **blemishes**. Known for its strong **antibacterial** and **antifungal** properties, tea tree oil helps to fight the bacteria that cause acne, reducing inflammation and preventing future breakouts. It also helps to calm **redness** and **swelling** in the skin. Tea tree oil can be applied topically (diluted with a carrier oil) to affected areas to help treat acne spots, or added to your daily skincare routine for a preventative approach.

Lavender Oil is another versatile essential oil that offers a range of benefits for the skin. Known for its **anti-inflammatory** and **healing** properties, lavender oil helps to soothe irritated skin, reduce redness, and promote the regeneration of skin cells. It is particularly effective for those dealing with **dry skin**, **eczema**, or **rosacea**. Lavender oil also supports wound healing and can reduce the appearance of **scars** or **stretch marks** when applied regularly. Its calming aroma also makes it a great choice for enhancing relaxation during your skincare routine.

Frankincense Oil, with its deep, earthy aroma, is widely used in skincare for its **anti-aging** benefits. Known for its ability to stimulate cell regeneration, frankincense oil helps to improve skin elasticity, reduce the appearance of fine lines and wrinkles, and promote overall skin tone. It also has **anti-inflammatory** properties, which can help calm irritated skin and reduce puffiness. Frankincense oil is especially useful for mature or aging skin and can be added to facial oils or creams to promote a youthful, glowing complexion.

For **dry skin** or **dehydration**, **Rosemary Oil** is an excellent choice. It is known for its ability to improve circulation, which helps to deliver nutrients and oxygen to the skin, promoting a healthier, more vibrant appearance. Rosemary oil is also rich in **antioxidants**, which help to fight free radicals and protect the skin from environmental stressors. It can be combined with a moisturizer or used in a facial steam to promote hydration and restore a youthful glow to dry skin.

Geranium Oil is another essential oil known for its ability to balance skin tone and improve elasticity. It is particularly beneficial for individuals with **oily skin** or **combination skin** because it helps regulate sebum production while maintaining moisture balance. Geranium oil also helps to promote blood circulation, which can reduce the appearance of **blemishes** and **dark spots**. Regular use of geranium oil can help to tone and tighten the skin, improving its overall texture and appearance.

For those dealing with **dark spots** or **hyperpigmentation**, **Lemon Oil** can be particularly beneficial. Lemon oil is known for its **brightening** properties and can help to lighten dark spots, age spots, and sun damage. It also has **antioxidant** and **antimicrobial** properties that protect the skin from environmental damage and promote an even skin tone. Lemon oil can be used in facial serums or added to a DIY face mask for a brightening boost. However, it's important to be cautious with lemon oil during the daytime, as it can cause **photosensitivity**, so it's best to use it in the evening or at night.

Chamomile Oil, particularly **Roman chamomile**, is well-known for its soothing properties. It is especially effective for calming **sensitive skin** and treating conditions like **eczema, rosacea**, and **rashes**. Chamomile oil has anti-inflammatory effects that help reduce irritation, redness, and itching. It also supports skin regeneration and healing, making it useful for treating dry, inflamed, or irritated skin. A few drops of chamomile oil can be added to a carrier oil and applied to sensitive areas to provide immediate relief.

For **scars** and **stretch marks**, **Helichrysum Oil** is an excellent essential oil to include in your skincare routine. Known for its **regenerative** and **healing** properties, helichrysum oil supports the repair of damaged skin and helps to reduce the appearance of scars and stretch marks. It promotes tissue regeneration and helps the skin heal faster, making it particularly beneficial for those with **post-surgical scars**, **acne scars**, or **stretch marks** from pregnancy or weight changes. Helichrysum oil can be diluted with a carrier oil and massaged into affected areas for best results.

Carrot Seed Oil is a powerful oil for promoting healthy, glowing skin. It is particularly beneficial for **dry**, **aging**, or **sun-damaged skin** due to its **regenerative** and **antioxidant** properties. Carrot seed oil helps stimulate collagen production, improving skin elasticity and reducing the appearance of fine lines and wrinkles. It also helps to repair **sun damage** and brighten the complexion, making it a great choice for individuals with **dull skin** or **uneven skin tone**.

Incorporating essential oils into your skincare routine can be done in a variety of ways. They can be diffused into the air to create a soothing environment or added to a **carrier oil** (such as coconut, jojoba, or almond oil) for topical application. You can also add essential oils to your favorite facial creams, body lotions, or bath products to enhance their benefits. Always ensure that you dilute essential oils properly before applying them to the skin to avoid irritation, and perform a patch test if using a new oil.

Aromatherapy offers a natural, effective way to care for your skin while reaping the additional benefits of emotional and physical well-being. By using the right essential oils, you can address a range of skin concerns and enhance the overall health of your skin, all while enjoying the calming and rejuvenating properties of essential oils.

Essential oils for Different Skin Types

Aromatherapy offers a wide variety of essential oils that can be tailored to suit different skin types, each with unique needs and concerns. These plant-derived oils contain bioactive compounds that can help soothe, hydrate, balance, and protect the skin. By selecting the right essential oils, you can address specific issues related to dryness, oiliness, sensitivity, or aging. Below are some of the best essential oils for each skin type, helping you create a customized skincare routine.

For Oily Skin:

Oily skin often results from overactive sebaceous glands that produce excess sebum. Essential oils for oily skin should focus on balancing oil production and preventing clogged pores.

- **Tea Tree Oil** is one of the most effective essential oils for oily skin. Its strong **antibacterial** and **antiseptic** properties help control acne breakouts by fighting the bacteria that cause pimples. Tea tree oil also helps regulate sebum production, making it ideal for oily or acne-prone skin. It can be applied directly to blemishes or mixed with a carrier oil for overall face application.
- **Lemon Oil** is another excellent choice for oily skin. It has natural **astringent** properties that help to tighten the skin and reduce excess oil. Lemon oil can also help brighten the complexion and reduce the appearance of acne scars or blemishes. However, it's important to use lemon oil with caution during the day, as it can make the skin sensitive to sunlight (photosensitive), so it's best used at night.
- **Geranium Oil** is useful for oily skin as it helps to balance sebum production while also maintaining the skin's moisture. It has **antibacterial** and **antifungal** properties, making it a good choice for preventing skin infections and promoting a healthy, clear complexion.

For Dry Skin:

Dry skin is often caused by a lack of moisture or dehydration, leaving the skin feeling tight and flaky. Essential oils for dry skin should focus on **hydration**, **nourishment**, and **regeneration**.

- **Lavender Oil** is known for its soothing and **moisturizing** properties. It helps to calm the skin, reduce inflammation, and support healing, making it perfect for dry, irritated skin. Lavender also promotes circulation and tissue regeneration, which can be beneficial for overall skin health.
- **Frankincense Oil** is a deeply hydrating essential oil that promotes cell regeneration and helps maintain skin elasticity. It works to rejuvenate and tone dry skin, improving texture and tone. Frankincense also has **anti-inflammatory** properties, which can reduce any redness or irritation associated with dryness.
- **Rose Oil**, particularly **Rose Otto**, is a luxurious oil with **moisturizing** and **anti-aging** properties. It helps restore moisture, improve skin texture, and reduce the appearance of fine lines. Rose oil also soothes dry, irritated skin and promotes a healthy, glowing complexion.
- **Carrot Seed Oil** is perfect for dry, aging skin. It helps rejuvenate and **hydrate** the skin while providing **antioxidant** protection. Carrot seed oil stimulates collagen production, helping to prevent wrinkles and maintain the skin's elasticity.

For Sensitive Skin:

Sensitive skin requires essential oils that are gentle, soothing, and calming. These oils help to reduce irritation, redness, and inflammation.

- **Chamomile Oil** (Roman chamomile) is known for its **anti-inflammatory** and **soothing** properties. It is perfect for sensitive skin, especially for conditions like **eczema**, **rosacea**, or **sunburn**. Chamomile oil helps reduce redness and irritation, providing a gentle way to calm inflammation and promote healing.
- **Helichrysum Oil** is another essential oil that can be beneficial for sensitive skin. Known for its healing and **anti-inflammatory** effects, helichrysum oil helps to regenerate tissue and repair damage, making it ideal for sensitive, reactive skin. It can also reduce the appearance of scars and promote a more even skin tone.
- **Lavender Oil** is not only great for dry skin but also for sensitive skin due to its calming and **anti-inflammatory** properties. It can soothe skin irritation, calm redness, and promote healing. Lavender oil is mild enough for sensitive skin and can be used daily to reduce sensitivity and discomfort.

For Mature Skin:

Mature or aging skin requires essential oils that promote **skin regeneration**, **hydration**, and **anti-aging** effects.

- **Rosemary Oil** is an excellent essential oil for promoting blood circulation, which in turn supports the health and vibrancy of mature skin. It has **antioxidant** properties that protect the skin from oxidative stress and free radical damage,

which contribute to the aging process. Rosemary also helps improve skin tone and elasticity, making it a valuable oil for mature skin.
- **Sandalwood Oil** is known for its **anti-aging** properties and ability to promote skin regeneration. It helps to **moisturize** and tighten the skin, reducing the appearance of fine lines and wrinkles. Sandalwood is particularly useful for promoting a youthful, glowing complexion and is gentle enough for daily use.
- **Frankincense Oil**, as mentioned earlier, is also highly beneficial for mature skin. It promotes the regeneration of skin cells, reduces the appearance of fine lines, and improves skin tone. Frankincense oil also stimulates the production of collagen, which helps maintain skin elasticity and smoothness.

For Combination Skin:

Combination skin often experiences both oily and dry patches, making it necessary to find essential oils that balance the skin's overall appearance and oil production.

- **Geranium Oil** is ideal for balancing combination skin. It helps regulate sebum production, ensuring that the skin doesn't become too oily while also providing moisture to dry areas. Geranium oil's **toning** and **anti-inflammatory** properties make it perfect for maintaining overall skin health and appearance.
- **Rosemary Oil** is also beneficial for combination skin as it helps to balance oil production without drying out the skin. It works to promote healthy circulation and can help tone and tighten the skin, reducing the appearance of both oily patches and dry spots.
- **Tea Tree Oil** can be added in small amounts to help control acne and oily skin areas without over-drying the skin. It helps combat bacteria while keeping the skin clear, but should be used in moderation to avoid irritation on drier areas of the face.

By choosing the right essential oils for your skin type, you can address specific skin concerns naturally while enjoying the therapeutic benefits of aromatherapy. Always remember to dilute essential oils with a carrier oil before applying them to the skin and perform a patch test to ensure there are no adverse reactions. With consistent use, these oils can help promote healthy, balanced skin that looks and feels its best.

Creating a Natural Skincare Routine with Essential Oils

A natural skincare routine incorporating essential oils can be a highly effective and luxurious way to nourish and care for your skin. Essential oils, with their potent healing properties, can target a variety of skin concerns, from acne and dryness to aging and irritation. By integrating these oils into a simple yet comprehensive skincare regimen, you can achieve healthy, glowing skin while also enjoying the therapeutic benefits of aromatherapy.

To start, it's essential to choose the right essential oils for your skin type and concerns. Essential oils work best when blended with a carrier oil, such as jojoba, coconut, or sweet almond oil, which helps to dilute their potent concentration and ensure they can be safely applied to the skin.

1. Cleansing:

A clean face is the foundation of any skincare routine. Instead of harsh chemical-based cleansers, you can use essential oils to create a gentle yet effective cleansing routine.

- **Tea Tree Oil** is ideal for acne-prone skin, as it has natural **antibacterial** and **antiseptic** properties. Add a few drops of tea tree oil to your facial cleanser or mix it with a carrier oil like jojoba oil to help prevent breakouts and cleanse the skin without stripping it of its natural oils.
- For **dry or sensitive skin**, **Lavender Oil** offers a soothing and calming cleanse. Its gentle, **anti-inflammatory** properties make it great for reducing irritation and redness, while still being effective at removing dirt and makeup. Mix a few drops with a gentle carrier oil and apply it to the face with a cotton pad to remove impurities.

2. Exfoliating:

Exfoliation is essential for removing dead skin cells and revealing a brighter, smoother complexion. Instead of using abrasive physical scrubs, essential oils can be added to natural exfoliants like sugar or coffee grounds to create a gentler, more nourishing scrub.

- **Frankincense Oil** helps to rejuvenate the skin by promoting cell regeneration. When mixed with a gentle exfoliating agent like brown sugar, frankincense oil can promote healthy skin turnover, reduce the appearance of fine lines, and stimulate collagen production. It is excellent for mature or aging skin.
- **Lemon Oil** has natural **astringent** and **brightening** properties. When combined with a sugar or sea salt scrub, it helps exfoliate dead skin while also lightening dark spots and evening out skin tone. Its **antioxidant** properties can also help protect the skin from environmental damage.

3. Toning:

Toners help to balance the skin's pH and tighten pores, providing a refreshing step in your skincare routine. Essential oils can help enhance the toning process, tightening and balancing skin tone while also offering additional benefits like hydration and healing.

- **Rosemary Oil** is great for toning oily or combination skin, as it helps to regulate sebum production and tighten the skin. It also has **antioxidant** properties that protect against free radical damage, making it perfect for those looking to maintain youthful, radiant skin.
- **Geranium Oil** is beneficial for **dry or sensitive skin**, as it helps to balance moisture levels while promoting skin regeneration. It can also help soothe irritated skin, reduce redness, and balance the skin's natural oils.

4. Moisturizing:

Moisturizing is a crucial step to keep the skin hydrated and supple. Essential oils can be incorporated into your moisturizer or used in a homemade blend to provide nourishment and hydration.

- **Jojoba Oil** is a great carrier oil for blending with essential oils, as its texture is similar to the skin's natural sebum. It works well for most skin types and helps to regulate oil production while providing moisture. Add a few drops of **Lavender Oil** or **Geranium Oil** to jojoba oil for a nourishing, balancing moisturizer.
- **Carrot Seed Oil** is rich in **vitamins** and **antioxidants**, making it an excellent choice for moisturizing dry, aging, or sun-damaged skin. It helps to improve skin elasticity and reduces the appearance of wrinkles and fine lines.

5. Spot Treatment:

For blemishes, acne, or other localized skin concerns, essential oils can be applied directly to the affected areas for targeted treatment.

- **Tea Tree Oil** is one of the most effective essential oils for treating **acne** and **blemishes**. Its antibacterial properties help kill acne-causing bacteria and reduce inflammation, promoting clear skin. Simply apply a diluted solution of tea tree oil to breakouts to prevent and treat acne.
- **Lavender Oil** is also beneficial for spot treatment, especially for calming inflammation and promoting healing. It can help reduce redness and swelling while preventing scarring, making it ideal for treating post-acne marks or irritated skin.

6. Hydration and Protection:

Nighttime skincare routines are essential for repairing and hydrating the skin while you sleep. Essential oils can help lock in moisture and promote skin repair overnight.

- **Chamomile Oil**, especially **Roman chamomile**, has anti-inflammatory and **soothing** effects, making it ideal for sensitive or irritated skin. Add a few drops to your evening moisturizer to calm and hydrate the skin overnight, helping to restore balance.
- **Sandalwood Oil** is deeply hydrating and helps with **skin regeneration**. Its **antioxidant** and **anti-inflammatory** properties help to reduce redness and irritation, making it perfect for rejuvenating the skin and fighting signs of aging. Sandalwood can be used in your nighttime routine to nourish and calm the skin while promoting relaxation.

7. Facial Masks:

Essential oils can also be used in homemade facial masks to provide additional treatment for specific skin concerns.

- **Clay masks** can be enhanced with **Lavender Oil** for a soothing, calming effect. Lavender helps to reduce skin irritation, clear acne, and balance oil production. Mix a few drops of lavender oil into a clay mask, along with honey or yogurt, for a hydrating, calming facial treatment.
- **Hyaluronic acid masks** can be infused with **Frankincense Oil** to promote skin regeneration and reduce the appearance of fine lines and wrinkles. Frankincense helps to stimulate cell turnover and supports healthy, glowing skin.

By incorporating essential oils into your daily skincare routine, you can address a wide range of skin concerns naturally while enhancing the overall health and vitality of your skin. Whether you're looking to balance oil production, reduce the appearance of aging, or soothe irritated skin, essential oils offer a safe and effective way to achieve a glowing, healthy complexion. Always remember to dilute essential oils properly with a carrier oil before applying to the skin, and perform a patch test to ensure compatibility with your skin type. With consistent use, essential oils can significantly enhance the effectiveness of your skincare routine, providing a natural, holistic approach to beauty.

Aromatherapy for Hair and Scalp Health

Aromatherapy offers a natural and effective approach to promoting hair and scalp health, using essential oils to address common concerns such as dryness, dandruff, hair thinning, and scalp irritation. These oils contain powerful plant-based compounds that can nourish, strengthen, and revitalize the hair and scalp, all while providing a relaxing, therapeutic experience. Incorporating essential oils into your hair care routine can help restore balance and vitality to your locks, naturally and safely.

For a healthy scalp and to promote hair growth, **Rosemary Oil** is one of the most popular essential oils. It has been shown to improve circulation to the scalp, stimulating the hair follicles and encouraging hair growth. Rosemary oil also helps balance oil production, making it ideal for both **oily** and **dry scalps**. Additionally, rosemary has **antioxidant** properties that help protect the scalp from free radical damage, which can lead to hair loss. Massaging rosemary oil into the scalp, diluted with a carrier oil such as jojoba or coconut oil, can help stimulate hair growth and reduce thinning over time.

Peppermint Oil is another excellent choice for boosting scalp health. Known for its cooling, invigorating properties, peppermint oil stimulates blood flow to the scalp, which can promote the growth of healthy, strong hair. The **menthol** in peppermint oil has an antimicrobial effect, which can help keep the scalp clean and free from **fungal** or **bacterial** infections that may lead to dandruff or scalp irritation. Its refreshing scent also provides a soothing and relaxing experience. To use, mix a few drops of peppermint oil with a carrier oil and massage gently into the scalp for a revitalizing treatment.

For dry scalp or **dandruff**, **Tea Tree Oil** is a powerful remedy. Tea tree oil is known for its **antifungal** and **antibacterial** properties, making it particularly effective for treating dandruff and **scalp infections** caused by yeast or bacteria. It helps clear away buildup of dead skin cells and flakes while soothing irritation and itchiness. Tea tree oil can be mixed with a carrier oil or added to a gentle shampoo to treat dandruff and maintain a healthy scalp.

Lavender Oil is not only great for relaxation but also beneficial for maintaining scalp health. Its **antibacterial** and **anti-inflammatory** properties help reduce scalp inflammation and irritation, which can contribute to hair thinning or shedding. Lavender oil also promotes hair growth by improving blood circulation to the scalp, ensuring that hair follicles receive the nutrients they need for optimal growth. A few drops of lavender oil can be added to your shampoo, conditioner, or a DIY hair mask for soothing and nourishing benefits.

For those looking to improve the overall health and strength of their hair, **Ylang-Ylang Oil** is an excellent choice. This floral-scented oil has been shown to balance oil production, making it suitable for both **oily** and **dry** hair types. Ylang-ylang oil helps promote a healthy scalp, strengthen hair strands, and improve hair texture. It can also help with **split ends** and **dryness** by promoting moisture retention in the hair. For best results, add a few drops of ylang-ylang oil to your conditioner or a hair mask, or dilute it in a carrier oil for a soothing scalp massage.

For **hair thinning** or **brittle hair**, **Cedarwood Oil** is particularly effective. It is thought to stimulate hair follicles by increasing circulation to the scalp, promoting **stronger** and **healthier** hair. Cedarwood oil is also known for balancing oil production, which is important for maintaining a clean and nourished scalp. It can be added to a carrier oil and massaged into the scalp or mixed into a shampoo for regular use to strengthen and protect hair from damage.

Lemon Oil is an excellent choice for cleansing the scalp and removing buildup from hair products, which can clog hair follicles and stunt hair growth. Its **astringent** properties help to balance the scalp's oil levels and clear away excess sebum, making it especially beneficial for those with oily scalps. Lemon oil also helps add shine and vitality to dull or lackluster hair. It can be diluted with a carrier oil or added to shampoo to enhance scalp health and improve hair's appearance.

Clary Sage Oil is another oil that can support overall hair health, especially for those experiencing hormonal imbalances that affect hair growth. It helps balance oil production in the scalp, promoting healthy hair and preventing scalp issues such as excessive dryness or oiliness. Clary sage oil also helps to improve hair texture, making it smoother and shinier. For best results, mix a few drops of clary sage oil with a carrier oil and massage into the scalp before rinsing.

To create a nourishing treatment for hair and scalp health, you can easily blend several essential oils together for a customized experience. For example, combining **rosemary**, **peppermint**, and **lavender** oils can help stimulate hair growth, reduce dandruff, and maintain a healthy, balanced scalp. You can mix these oils with a carrier oil and gently massage them into your scalp for several minutes, allowing the oils to absorb before rinsing. This treatment can be repeated 1-2 times per week for best results.

Using essential oils in your hair care routine is simple and effective. They can be applied directly to the scalp with a carrier oil, added to shampoos or conditioners, or used in hair masks to address a variety of hair and scalp concerns. Whether you are looking to promote hair growth, fight dandruff, balance oil production, or improve overall hair texture, aromatherapy provides a natural, non-invasive way to enhance scalp health and achieve beautiful, vibrant hair. Just be sure to dilute essential oils properly before use and perform a patch test to ensure compatibility with your skin.

Essential oils beneficial for hair and scalp

Essential oils are a natural and effective way to enhance hair and scalp health. These concentrated plant extracts contain powerful properties that can address a range of common concerns, from promoting hair growth to reducing dandruff and soothing scalp irritation. By incorporating the right essential oils into your hair care routine, you can nourish your scalp, improve hair texture, and achieve healthier, more vibrant hair.

Rosemary Oil is one of the most popular essential oils for hair care. It is known for stimulating blood circulation to the scalp, which helps nourish hair follicles and promote hair growth. Rosemary oil is particularly beneficial for people experiencing **hair thinning** or **balding**, as it strengthens hair and helps prevent further hair loss. Additionally, rosemary oil has **antioxidant** properties that protect the scalp from free radical damage. It can be mixed with a carrier oil like jojoba or coconut oil and massaged into the scalp for a revitalizing treatment that promotes both scalp health and hair growth.

Lavender Oil is not only calming but also has multiple benefits for hair. It helps improve blood circulation to the scalp, which can stimulate hair follicles and promote the growth of healthy, thick hair. Lavender oil is especially effective for those dealing with **scalp inflammation**, **itchiness**, or **dryness**, thanks to its **soothing** and **anti-inflammatory** properties. It is also known to balance oil production, making it suitable for both dry and oily scalps. A few drops of lavender oil can be added to a carrier oil for a relaxing scalp massage or included in a DIY hair mask.

Peppermint Oil is another essential oil that is invigorating and beneficial for the scalp. The **menthol** in peppermint oil helps stimulate circulation to the scalp, which can promote hair growth and improve overall scalp health. Peppermint oil also has a **cooling** and **refreshing** effect, which can soothe **itchiness** and inflammation. This oil is particularly beneficial for those with **oily scalps** since it helps regulate oil production while maintaining hydration. For best results, dilute peppermint oil with a carrier oil and gently massage it into the scalp before rinsing.

Tea Tree Oil is renowned for its **antibacterial**, **antifungal**, and **antiseptic** properties, making it highly effective in combating scalp conditions such as dandruff, **itchiness**, and **fungal infections**. Tea tree oil can help clear away scalp buildup, remove flakes, and soothe irritated skin. It's especially beneficial for those dealing with dandruff or

seborrheic dermatitis. Tea tree oil can be added to your regular shampoo or mixed with a carrier oil and massaged directly into the scalp to restore balance and prevent infection.

Cedarwood Oil is an excellent option for improving scalp circulation and reducing dandruff. It has **antifungal** and **antibacterial** properties, which help address scalp issues and maintain a healthy scalp environment. Cedarwood oil can also help regulate oil production, making it a suitable choice for people with **dry** or **oily** scalps. By improving blood flow to the scalp, cedarwood oil supports hair growth and strengthens the hair roots, helping to prevent hair thinning and breakage. It can be used as part of a scalp massage or added to a shampoo for added benefits.

Ylang-Ylang Oil is particularly beneficial for individuals with dry or brittle hair. This essential oil helps to balance the scalp's oil production, providing hydration without making the scalp greasy. Ylang-ylang oil has a nurturing effect on the hair and scalp, helping to prevent **split ends**, **hair thinning**, and **dryness**. The moisturizing properties of ylang-ylang help restore the hair's natural shine and strength. You can add ylang-ylang oil to a DIY hair mask or mix it with a carrier oil and massage it gently into the scalp to enhance hydration and promote healthier hair.

Clary Sage Oil is great for improving scalp health and promoting hair growth. It has **antioxidant** properties that protect hair from environmental damage and help to balance oil production on the scalp. Clary sage oil is also known to regulate hormones, making it particularly effective for individuals experiencing **hormonal imbalances** that affect hair health. It can be used to treat **dry scalp**, **brittle hair**, and hair loss. Clary sage oil can be added to shampoos, conditioners, or massaged into the scalp with a carrier oil to help maintain balance and stimulate hair growth.

Bergamot Oil, derived from the rind of the bergamot orange, is often used to improve scalp health by reducing dandruff and promoting hair strength. Bergamot oil has **antibacterial** properties that help cleanse the scalp, preventing buildup and keeping the hair follicles clean. It also helps with **oily scalp** issues by balancing sebum production. The uplifting aroma of bergamot oil can also have a calming effect, making it a great addition to your hair care routine for both physical and emotional well-being.

Lemon Oil is known for its ability to balance the scalp's oil levels and promote a clean, refreshed feeling. It has **astringent** properties, which help tighten the skin on the scalp and reduce excess oil production. Lemon oil also has **antibacterial** properties that help keep the scalp free from infection and buildup, which can lead to hair loss. It also helps brighten hair, giving it a natural shine and healthy appearance. Lemon oil can be added to your shampoo or diluted in a carrier oil for a scalp massage.

Using essential oils for hair and scalp health is a simple yet effective way to enhance your hair care routine. Whether you're looking to promote hair growth, prevent dandruff, balance oil production, or improve the overall health of your hair, these oils offer a natural solution. Always remember to dilute essential oils with a carrier oil, such as jojoba, argan, or coconut oil, to avoid skin irritation. Regular use of essential oils can provide long-term benefits for a healthy scalp and stronger, shinier hair.

Crafting Haircare Products with Essential Oils

Crafting your own haircare products with essential oils is a rewarding and natural way to promote healthy hair and scalp. These oils are packed with beneficial properties that can address a wide range of hair concerns, such as dryness, dandruff, oiliness, and thinning hair. By combining essential oils with simple, natural ingredients like carrier oils, herbs, and natural clays, you can create effective, personalized treatments tailored to your specific hair type and needs.

When crafting haircare products, it's essential to choose the right **essential oils** based on your hair and scalp concerns. These concentrated oils can be used in **shampoos, conditioners, hair masks**, and **scalp treatments**. The key to creating an effective product is to blend essential oils with appropriate **carrier oils** and other natural ingredients that complement their properties.

Shampoo

Making a natural, essential oil-infused shampoo is simple and highly effective. Start with a base of mild, **natural shampoo** or liquid castile soap, and then add essential oils to target your specific hair concerns.

- **Tea Tree Oil** is an excellent addition for oily or dandruff-prone scalps. Its **antibacterial** and **antifungal** properties help cleanse the scalp, prevent infections, and clear away flakes.
- **Lavender Oil** is ideal for soothing the scalp, reducing itchiness, and promoting healthy hair growth. Its calming effect also reduces scalp irritation and inflammation.
- **Peppermint Oil** is a great choice for invigorating the scalp and improving circulation, which helps promote hair growth. It also adds a refreshing scent and tingly sensation.

To craft your own shampoo, combine 1/4 cup of liquid castile soap with 10-15 drops of your chosen essential oils. Adjust the essential oil quantities based on your preference for scent or intensity. This blend can be stored in a bottle and used as you would any regular shampoo.

Conditioner

Conditioners infused with essential oils provide nourishment and moisture while promoting healthy hair. Start with a natural, unscented conditioner base, and add essential oils that support hydration, shine, and scalp health.

- **Geranium Oil** works well for balancing oil production in both dry and oily hair types, making it an excellent choice for those with combination hair.
- **Ylang-Ylang Oil** is a great moisturizing oil for dry, brittle hair. It helps to restore the natural shine and softness of hair by improving moisture retention.
- **Rosemary Oil** can help stimulate circulation to the scalp, which may encourage hair growth while providing shine and vitality to the hair shaft.

To make your own conditioner, mix 1/4 cup of a natural, unscented conditioner with 10-15 drops of essential oils. Apply to damp hair after shampooing, leave for a few minutes and rinse thoroughly.

Hair Masks

Hair masks provide deep conditioning and nourishment, making them an excellent treatment for dry or damaged hair. Essential oils can be blended into a base of hydrating ingredients like honey, yogurt, or avocado to create a rich, restorative mask.

- **Avocado Oil** is a rich source of vitamins and fatty acids, which help hydrate and strengthen the hair. Combine it with **Lavender Oil** or **Frankincense Oil** to soothe a dry or irritated scalp.
- **Honey**, with its natural humectant properties, helps lock in moisture. Adding **Rosemary Oil** and **Tea Tree Oil** can help stimulate the scalp and reduce dandruff.

To make a nourishing hair mask, combine 1/4 cup of avocado or coconut oil with 1 tablespoon of honey. Add 10-15 drops of essential oils like **Rosemary** or **Lavender**. Apply the mask generously to damp hair, cover with a shower cap, and leave for 20-30 minutes before rinsing.

Scalp Treatments

Regular scalp treatments with essential oils can help maintain a healthy, balanced scalp, which is crucial for strong hair growth. Essential oils can help remove buildup, balance oil production, and improve circulation to the hair follicles.

- **Cedarwood Oil** promotes circulation, helping to nourish hair follicles and encourage hair growth. It's particularly helpful for individuals with **thinning hair**

- **Lemon Oil** helps cleanse the scalp by removing excess oils and product buildup. Its **astringent** properties help tighten the skin, which can balance oil production and reduce dandruff.
- **Chamomile Oil** soothes the scalp and reduces inflammation, making it perfect for sensitive skin or irritated scalps.

To create a scalp treatment, mix 2 tablespoons of a carrier oil like **jojoba** or **coconut oil** with 5-10 drops of your chosen essential oils. Massage this mixture gently into the scalp, leave for about 20 minutes, and then wash with a mild shampoo.

Hair Growth Serum

For those looking to stimulate hair growth or prevent hair loss, essential oils can be combined into a growth serum to nourish and energize the scalp.

- **Rosemary Oil** is widely recognized for promoting hair growth by stimulating circulation to the scalp.
- **Peppermint Oil** promotes circulation and has a refreshing, stimulating effect on the scalp that can promote healthier hair.
- **Lavender Oil** promotes relaxation and supports a healthy scalp environment conducive to hair growth.

Combine 2 tablespoons of **castor oil** (which is known to support hair growth) with 5-10 drops of **Rosemary** and **Peppermint** oils. Massage the serum into your scalp every few days, focusing on areas where hair is thinning, and leave for 30 minutes before rinsing.

Shine-Enhancing Spray

To add natural shine and protect your hair from environmental damage, you can craft a shine-enhancing hair spray. Essential oils like **Geranium** and **Lavender** can be used to balance moisture and add a soft, healthy shine.

- **Geranium Oil** helps promote balance in both oily and dry hair types, enhancing overall texture and giving hair a glossy finish.
- **Lemon Oil** adds a natural shine and helps clarify hair, making it appear brighter and more vibrant.

To make a shine spray, mix 1 cup of distilled water with 10-15 drops of essential oils, such as **Geranium** or **Lemon**. Pour into a spray bottle and lightly mist onto hair for a refreshing and glossy finish.

Important Tips for Crafting Haircare Products:

1. **Patch Test**: Before applying any DIY haircare product, conduct a patch test to ensure you don't have any allergic reactions or irritation from the essential oils.
2. **Dilution**: Always dilute essential oils with a carrier oil (like jojoba, almond, or coconut oil) to prevent irritation, especially when using them on the scalp or hair.
3. **Storage**: Keep your homemade haircare products in dark glass containers to protect the oils from light, which can degrade their quality.
4. **Consistency**: For the best results, use your homemade haircare products consistently. Natural treatments may take a few weeks to show visible changes, s patience is key.

By crafting your own haircare products with essential oils, you can address specific concerns, create a personalized routine, and enjoy the natural benefits of aromatherapy for your hair and scalp health. Whether you're seeking to promote growth, balance oil production, or simply enhance the shine of your hair, essential oils offer an effective and enjoyable way to nurture your hair from root to tip.

Creating an Aromatherapy Massage at Home

Aromatherapy massage is a wonderful way to relax and promote both physical and emotional well-being, and you don't have to go to a spa to enjoy its benefits. By incorporating essential oils into your massage routine, you can enhance relaxation, reduce muscle tension, and uplift your mood right in the comfort of your home. The combination of soothing touch and therapeutic oils helps to relieve stress, improve circulation, and rejuvenate the body and mind.

To start, you'll need a few key items: **carrier oils**, **essential oils**, and a comfortable space to unwind. Carrier oils are essential for diluting the potent essential oils and ensuring they are safe for application on the skin. Popular choices include **jojoba oil, sweet almond oil, coconut oil**, and **grapeseed oil**. These oils are lightweight and absorb easily into the skin, providing the perfect base for your essential oil blend.

Choosing the Right Essential Oils

The essential oils you choose will depend on the therapeutic effects you want to achieve. Below are some popular options, each with unique benefits:

- **Lavender Oil** is one of the most versatile and widely used oils for relaxation. It has **calming**, **anti-inflammatory**, and **muscle-relaxing** properties that make it ideal for relieving tension, promoting sleep, and soothing the mind. Lavender oil is perfect for unwinding after a long day or for reducing stress before bedtime.
- **Peppermint Oil** is invigorating and refreshing, offering **cooling** and **pain-relieving** effects. It is often used to ease **muscle soreness**, headaches, and digestive issues. The **menthol** in peppermint oil stimulates circulation, which can enhance energy levels and ease tight muscles, making it an excellent choice for a pre-workout massage or a revitalizing treatment.
- **Eucalyptus Oil** is known for its **decongestant** properties, making it great for respiratory support. It helps clear the airways, making it an ideal oil for use during a massage when you're feeling under the weather or dealing with **sinus congestion**. It also has **analgesic** properties that help relieve joint and muscle pain.
- **Sweet Orange Oil** is uplifting and bright, perfect for improving mood and boosting energy levels. The **citrusy** aroma of orange oil can help alleviate feelings of stress and anxiety while providing a refreshing, joyful atmosphere during your

massage. It's a great oil to use when you're feeling low or in need of a little emotional boost.
- **Frankincense Oil** is deeply grounding and known for its ability to promote relaxation and **spiritual well-being**. It is often used to ease stress and promote emotional balance. Frankincense also has **anti-inflammatory** properties, making it helpful for joint pain and stiffness.

Preparing Your Aromatherapy Massage Blend

Now that you've chosen your essential oils, the next step is to mix them with a carrier oil. This is important because essential oils are highly concentrated, and using them directly on the skin can cause irritation. A safe ratio is generally 1-2 drops of essential oil per teaspoon of carrier oil for general use. If you're doing a more targeted treatment, such as for sore muscles, you can increase the number of drops slightly, but always keep within safe dilution levels.

For a **relaxing massage**, you might try the following blend:

- 1 tablespoon of **sweet almond oil**
- 3 drops of **lavender oil**
- 2 drops of **frankincense oil**

For a **refreshing and invigorating massage**, use:

- 1 tablespoon of **jojoba oil**
- 3 drops of **peppermint oil**
- 2 drops of **eucalyptus oil**

For a **mood-boosting massage**, you can blend:

- 1 tablespoon of **coconut oil**
- 3 drops of **sweet orange oil**
- 2 drops of **lavender oil**

Setting Up Your Space

Creating a relaxing environment is key to enhancing the benefits of your aromatherapy massage. Begin by ensuring you have a quiet, comfortable area with minimal distractions. Light some **candles**, use soft lighting, and play relaxing **music** to set the mood. If possible, use a **massage table** or a comfortable surface like a soft bed or mat to lay on. Warm the room to a comfortable temperature to help you fully relax during the massage.

you have a partner or friend helping with the massage, ensure that the person giving the massage knows which areas of your body require attention and how much pressure to apply. You can also perform a self-massage on areas like the neck, shoulders, hands, or feet, where tension often builds up.

Massage Techniques

When applying the oil blend, use smooth, firm strokes to encourage relaxation and relieve muscle tension. Here are some techniques to consider:

- **Effleurage**: Gentle, gliding strokes used to warm up the muscles and promote relaxation. This technique is especially useful for the back and shoulders.
- **Petrissage**: Kneading movements, ideal for massaging the **neck, shoulders**, or **legs** to help release tension and improve circulation.
- **Circular Movements**: Use your fingertips to make small circles on areas where tension is concentrated, such as the **temples, jawline**, or **lower back**.
- **Tapping**: Light tapping movements can help invigorate the body and stimulate circulation, especially useful for areas like the arms and legs.

Enjoying the Full Benefits

For the most benefit, allow the essential oils to absorb into your skin and continue their soothing effects after the massage. Drink plenty of water afterward to help flush out any toxins that may have been released from your muscles. Afterward, allow your body to rest and absorb the relaxation and healing benefits of the essential oils.

Regularly practicing aromatherapy massage at home is a wonderful way to relieve stress, improve circulation, and nourish the body and mind. Whether used to soothe aching muscles, improve sleep, or uplift the spirit, the combination of massage and essential oils creates a deeply relaxing and therapeutic experience that promotes overall wellness.

Selecting the Right Carrier Oils

Choosing the right carrier oil is a crucial step in the safe and effective use of essential oils in aromatherapy. Carrier oils serve as the base for diluting concentrated essential oils, allowing them to be safely applied to the skin. They also provide their own unique benefits, such as hydration, nourishment, and skin protection. With so many options available, it's important to select the right carrier oil for your skin type, personal preferences, and the specific therapeutic effects you are seeking.

1. Jojoba Oil

Jojoba oil is one of the most commonly used carrier oils in aromatherapy due to its similarity to the skin's natural sebum. It's an excellent choice for most skin types, especially for those with **oily** or **acne-prone skin**, as it helps regulate oil production without clogging pores. Jojoba oil is lightweight, non-greasy, and absorbs quickly into the skin. It also has moisturizing properties and helps to balance the skin's hydration, making it suitable for **dry** or **combination skin** as well. Its mild nature makes it a great option for use on the face and body.

2. Sweet Almond Oil

Sweet almond oil is a rich, nourishing oil that is ideal for **dry** or **sensitive skin**. Packed with vitamins A, E, and D, this carrier oil is known for its ability to soften and hydrate the skin. It's gentle enough for use on delicate skin areas, such as the face, and is often used to help improve the appearance of **dry patches**, **scarring**, and **stretch marks**. Sweet almond oil has a mild, nutty scent that blends well with most essential oils, making it a versatile choice for creating massage blends or adding to skin care formulations.

3. Coconut Oil

Coconut oil is highly prized for its **moisturizing** and **antibacterial** properties. It is particularly beneficial for **dry skin** or **flaky scalp** conditions. With its high content of fatty acids, coconut oil can deeply hydrate the skin and protect it from moisture loss. It also has a pleasant, tropical scent and is commonly used in hair care products to treat **dry hair** and **split ends**. However, since coconut oil is comedogenic for some people, those with **oily skin** or **acne-prone skin** should use it cautiously and test for sensitivity.

4. Grapeseed Oil

Grapeseed oil is a light, non-greasy oil that is packed with antioxidants, including vitamin E. It is an excellent choice for **oily** or **acne-prone skin**, as it helps to regulate oil production and has **astringent** properties that can help tighten and tone the skin. Grapeseed oil is easily absorbed, making it perfect for those who prefer a lightweight, non-clogging option. It's also rich in linoleic acid, which can help strengthen the skin's barrier and reduce the appearance of scars and blemishes.

5. Argan Oil

Argan oil is a luxurious, rich oil that is ideal for **mature**, **dry**, or **damaged skin**. Known for its high content of essential fatty acids, antioxidants, and vitamin E, argan oil deeply nourishes and repairs the skin. It's especially effective at reducing **fine lines** and promoting skin elasticity. Argan oil also works wonders for dry, **frizzy hair**, as it helps to restore moisture and shine. Its lightweight nature and quick absorption make it suitable for use on the face and body, making it a popular choice in anti-aging skin care.

6. Olive Oil

Olive oil is a widely available carrier oil that is packed with vitamins, minerals, and antioxidants. It is highly moisturizing and can benefit **dry** or **mature skin** by replenishing lost moisture and promoting a youthful glow. Olive oil also has soothing properties and is often used to treat irritated or inflamed skin. While it is heavier than some other oils, its rich texture is perfect for dry or aging skin, but it may be too thick for those with **oily** or **sensitive skin**.

7. Avocado Oil

Avocado oil is a deeply nourishing oil that is perfect for **dry**, **mature**, or **sun-damaged skin**. Rich in vitamins A, D, and E, as well as fatty acids, avocado oil helps to hydrate and repair the skin. It's also known for its ability to improve skin elasticity and promote collagen production, making it an excellent choice for anti-aging formulations. Because it's a heavier oil, avocado oil works best when used in targeted treatments, such as on the face or areas of the body that are prone to dryness and wrinkles.

8. Rosehip Seed Oil

Rosehip seed oil is a lightweight, non-greasy oil known for its ability to regenerate the skin. It is packed with essential fatty acids, vitamin C, and antioxidants, making it an excellent choice for treating **sun damage**, **scars**, and **hyperpigmentation**. Rosehip oil helps stimulate collagen production, which can improve skin texture and reduce the appearance of wrinkles. It's often recommended for **aging skin**, and its ability to improve skin tone and texture makes it ideal for those dealing with **uneven skin tone** or **blemishes**.

9. Castor Oil

Castor oil is known for its **thick**, **viscous** texture and is often used for promoting hair growth and treating **dry scalp**. It is rich in **ricinoleic acid**, which helps improve circulation and support hair follicle health. When used as a scalp treatment, castor oil can help reduce **hair thinning** and promote **stronger hair growth**. While castor oil is best known for its use in hair care, it can also be beneficial for dry or cracked skin, as it deeply hydrates and promotes healing.

10. Hemp Seed Oil

Hemp seed oil is an excellent carrier oil for **sensitive** and **inflammatory skin** conditions. It has a perfect balance of omega-3 and omega-6 fatty acids, making it incredibly nourishing for the skin. Hemp seed oil is non-comedogenic, meaning it won't clog pores, and it can help regulate oil production. It's also known for its ability to reduce **redness** and **inflammation**, making it a great option for individuals dealing with **eczema**, **rosacea**, or **acne**.

How to Choose the Right Carrier Oil:

1. **Consider Your Skin Type**: Choose a carrier oil that matches your skin's needs. For dry or mature skin, opt for richer oils like **argan** or **avocado**. For oily or acne prone skin, **jojoba**, **grapeseed**, or **hemp seed** oil may be better options.
2. **Pay Attention to the Scent**: Some carrier oils, such as **coconut oil**, have a distinct scent, while others, like **jojoba** or **grapeseed**, have little to no fragrance. Choose an oil that complements the scent of your essential oils.
3. **Consider the Oil's Texture**: Lighter oils, such as **grapeseed** or **jojoba**, absorb quickly and are ideal for those who prefer a non-greasy finish. Heavier oils like **olive** or **avocado** are better for targeted treatments on dry skin.
4. **Patch Test**: Always conduct a patch test when trying a new carrier oil to ensure you don't have an allergic reaction or sensitivity to it.

By selecting the right carrier oil for your skin type and concerns, you can create personalized, effective aromatherapy blends that nourish your skin while reaping the benefits of essential oils. Each carrier oil brings unique properties that can enhance the effectiveness of your chosen essential oils, providing the ultimate holistic skincare experience.

Techniques for a Relaxing Aromatherapy Massage

Aromatherapy massage is a deeply relaxing and therapeutic experience that combines the soothing effects of essential oils with the physical benefits of massage. This holistic practice not only helps relieve tension in the muscles but also promotes emotional well-being by calming the mind, reducing stress, and enhancing mood. By using the right techniques, you can maximize the therapeutic benefits of aromatherapy oils and create a serene, healing environment.

Preparing for the Massage

Before beginning the massage, it's essential to create a calming environment. Choose a quiet, comfortable space with soft lighting, soothing music, and a pleasant aroma. You can use candles or a diffuser to help disperse your chosen essential oils into the air, setting the mood for the session. If you're using a diffuser, consider oils like **lavender** or **chamomile** for a relaxing atmosphere. It's also important to make sure the room is warm, as this will help the muscles relax and allow the oils to be absorbed more effectively.

Choosing the Right Essential Oils

The essential oils you choose will play a key role in the overall effectiveness of the massage. Select oils based on the desired outcome—whether it's to relieve physical tension, promote relaxation, or uplift the mood.

- For **relaxation** and stress relief, **lavender** and **chamomile** are excellent choices.
- For **muscle relaxation** and pain relief, **peppermint**, **eucalyptus**, and **rosemary** can be particularly effective.
- For a **mood boost**, citrus oils like **orange** and **bergamot** are uplifting and refreshing.

Dilute the essential oils in a carrier oil, such as **jojoba**, **sweet almond**, or **coconut oil**, which will ensure that the essential oils are safe to apply directly to the skin while also providing nourishment and hydration.

Massage Techniques

The techniques you use during the massage will influence how deeply the oils are absorbed into the skin and how effective the relaxation process is. Below are several techniques to incorporate into your aromatherapy massage for maximum benefit:

Effleurage (Long, Gliding Strokes)

Effleurage is a foundational technique in aromatherapy massage, involving smooth, long gliding strokes along the body. This technique is great for promoting relaxation, warming up the muscles, and preparing the body for deeper work. Use the palms of your hands to apply gentle pressure, moving from the neck and shoulders down to the back, arms, and legs. Effleurage helps stimulate circulation, allowing the essential oils to penetrate the skin effectively.

- Start at the shoulders and move toward the arms or back in long, flowing motions
- Apply moderate pressure, adjusting based on the comfort level of the person receiving the massage.

Petrissage (Kneading)

Petrissage involves kneading the muscles with the fingers or palms, and it is especially useful for releasing deep tension and tightness in the muscles. This technique can be applied to larger muscle groups, such as the back, thighs, and calves. It helps to increase circulation, relieve muscle soreness, and promote relaxation.

- Gently lift and knead the muscles between your fingers or palms, applying deeper pressure as needed.
- Focus on areas where tension is more concentrated, such as the shoulders or lower back.

Tapotement (Rhythmic Tapping)

Tapotement involves rhythmic tapping or percussion using the edge of your hands or fingers. This technique stimulates the muscles and promotes blood flow, offering a refreshing, invigorating sensation. It's particularly helpful for people feeling fatigued or in need of a pick-me-up. It's also used to stimulate the nerves, improve circulation, and relieve congestion.

- Use your fingertips or the edge of your hands to tap lightly on the body in quick succession.
- Avoid applying too much pressure; the movement should be gentle but firm enough to stimulate the skin.

Friction (Circular Movements)

...riction involves using circular movements to generate heat and penetrate deeper into the muscles. This technique is great for loosening knots or tight areas, especially in the neck, shoulders, and lower back. Applying firm, circular pressure helps stimulate the tissue, increase circulation, and aid in the absorption of essential oils.

- Apply moderate pressure with your thumbs or fingertips and use small, circular motions over tense areas.
- Focus on areas with tight muscles or knots, working the oil into the skin.

Vibration (Shaking Movements)

Vibration involves gently shaking the muscles with a quick, rhythmic movement. This technique is particularly effective for relieving muscle tightness and promoting relaxation. It's useful for areas with tension, such as the neck, back, or thighs. Vibration helps release deep muscle tension and enhance the soothing effects of the oils.

- Use a light shaking motion with your hands or fingertips, applying minimal pressure.
- Focus on areas where the muscles feel tight or sore, such as the shoulders or upper back.

Pressure Points and Targeted Focus

Incorporating pressure point techniques into your aromatherapy massage can enhance the relaxation experience. Apply gentle pressure to key points along the body, such as the temples, the area between the eyebrows, or the base of the skull, to help release tension. This can also help promote mental clarity, reduce headaches, and improve overall relaxation.

- For **headaches** or **sinus congestion**, gently press the area between the eyebrows or the temples, using small circular motions.
- For **stress relief**, focus on the back of the neck and the shoulders, which are common areas for tension accumulation.

Finishing the Massage

To finish the massage, use slow, sweeping strokes to help relax the muscles and calm the mind. Gradually reduce the pressure and focus on using lighter strokes to bring the body back to a state of calm. This helps the oils to be absorbed fully into the skin, while also signaling the body that the massage is coming to an end.

Aftercare

After the aromatherapy massage, allow the oils to remain on the skin for at least 30 minutes to an hour, as they continue to work their healing properties. Drink plenty of water to help flush out toxins that may have been released during the massage. Relax and avoid strenuous activities to fully absorb the calming effects of the oils.

By combining these techniques with the power of essential oils, an aromatherapy massage becomes a deeply restorative experience for both the body and mind. Whether you are relieving tension, improving circulation, or boosting your mood, the right techniques and oils can offer profound relaxation and healing in the comfort of your own home.

Aromatherapy for Mindfulness and Meditation

Aromatherapy can be a powerful tool to enhance mindfulness and meditation, creating an environment that promotes relaxation, focus, and emotional balance. The use of essential oils in these practices helps deepen the meditative experience, support emotional clarity, and foster a sense of inner peace. By incorporating essential oils into your mindfulness and meditation routines, you can enhance your ability to remain present, calm your mind, and cultivate a deeper connection to your practice.

Choosing the Right Essential Oils for Meditation

Certain essential oils are particularly effective in promoting relaxation, grounding, and mental clarity, making them ideal companions for meditation. Selecting oils that align with the goals of your practice—whether it's calming the mind, improving focus, or fostering a sense of balance—can greatly enhance your meditation experience.

- **Frankincense Oil** is one of the most revered oils for meditation. Its grounding, calming properties help quiet the mind, reduce stress, and facilitate deeper states of meditation. Frankincense has been used in spiritual practices for centuries and is known for its ability to enhance the feeling of connection during meditation, helping you achieve a deeper sense of presence and awareness.
- **Lavender Oil** is widely recognized for its calming and soothing effects on the mind and body. It helps reduce anxiety, promote relaxation, and relieve mental tension. Lavender oil is particularly useful for those looking to quiet racing thoughts during meditation and achieve a peaceful state of mind. Its gentle aroma can help create a serene atmosphere conducive to mindful breathing and deep reflection.
- **Sandalwood Oil** is another excellent choice for mindfulness and meditation. It has a deep, woody aroma that promotes grounding, relaxation, and emotional clarity. Sandalwood is often used to enhance focus and encourage a peaceful state of mind, making it ideal for meditation practices that require concentration and mental clarity. Its soothing properties also help reduce feelings of anxiety and mental clutter.
- **Cedarwood Oil** has a warm, earthy scent that helps promote relaxation and stability, making it an excellent oil for grounding during meditation. Cedarwood is

known for its ability to calm the nervous system, reduce anxiety, and encourage emotional balance, helping you stay focused and centered throughout your practice.
- **Bergamot Oil** is uplifting and balancing, making it ideal for those who struggle with low mood or emotional imbalance. It is often used to promote feelings of joy, peace, and self-acceptance, making it particularly beneficial for meditation practices focused on self-reflection and emotional healing. Bergamot oil helps to lift the spirit, reduce stress, and create a sense of calm and harmony.

Using Aromatherapy to Enhance Mindfulness

Incorporating aromatherapy into mindfulness practice can enhance your ability to stay present and aware. The gentle scent of essential oils acts as an anchor, drawing your attention back to the present moment and helping you maintain focus. Aromatherapy can also deepen your sensory experience during mindfulness, allowing you to be more attuned to your body, breath, and surroundings.

- **Inhalation**: Simply inhaling essential oils can be an effective way to calm the mind and promote mindfulness. Using a diffuser is a convenient way to disperse the oils into the air, creating an aromatic environment that supports focus and relaxation. For a deeper effect, place a few drops of your chosen essential oil on a cotton ball or in the palm of your hands, and take slow, deep breaths. As you inhale, allow the aroma to guide you into the present moment, calming your mind and enhancing your sensory awareness.
- **Topical Application**: Applying essential oils directly to the skin can also help integrate aromatherapy into your mindfulness practice. Dilute the essential oil in a carrier oil, such as **jojoba** or **sweet almond oil**, and apply it to pulse points (wrists, temples, behind the ears) or areas of tension, such as the neck and shoulders. The calming aroma will serve as a reminder to return to the present moment, while the physical sensation of the oil on the skin can deepen your connection to your body.

Aromatherapy During Guided Meditation

Essential oils can enhance the experience of guided meditation by helping you stay focused and aligned with the practice. For example, using **lavender** or **frankincense** can create a calm atmosphere that reduces distractions and encourages deep relaxation. You can either diffuse the oils in the room or apply them topically before beginning the meditation.

If you're practicing a meditation technique that focuses on **breathwork**, try using **peppermint oil**, which can help open the airways and promote clear, deep breathing. This can enhance your ability to connect with your breath and stay present throughout the session. **Eucalyptus oil** is another good option for breath-focused meditation, as it helps clear the respiratory system and invigorate the mind.

Creating an Aromatherapy Meditation Ritual

For a more immersive aromatherapy meditation experience, you can develop a ritual that incorporates essential oils. Begin by selecting your essential oils and preparing your space. Use a diffuser to fill the room with the scent of your chosen oils, or light a scented candle with essential oils to create a calming ambiance. As you settle into your meditation space, take a few moments to breathe deeply and allow the aroma of the oils to wash over you.

Before you begin your meditation, you may want to anoint yourself with essential oils, applying them to your pulse points or chakra points. This ritual can help signal to your body and mind that you are entering a time of quiet reflection, making it easier to transition into a meditative state.

Combining Aromatherapy with Mindfulness Practices

In addition to meditation, aromatherapy can be paired with other mindfulness practices, such as yoga, Tai Chi, or walking meditation. Essential oils can enhance your focus, improve your mood, and support relaxation during these activities.

- **Yoga**: Using essential oils like **cedarwood, frankincense,** or **sandalwood** during your yoga practice can enhance grounding and improve focus during poses. The oils can help deepen your breath and create a calm atmosphere that encourages mindfulness in each movement.
- **Walking Meditation**: When walking in nature or practicing mindful walking, using oils like **lemon, bergamot,** or **peppermint** can invigorate your senses and heighten your awareness of your surroundings. Applying essential oils to your wrists or inhaling them as you walk can help you stay present and connected to your environment.

Conclusion

Aromatherapy is a powerful tool for enhancing mindfulness and meditation practices. Whether you're seeking relaxation, emotional clarity, or improved focus, the right essential oils can deepen your connection to the present moment and support your mental and emotional well-being. By selecting oils that align with your goals, incorporating them into your practice, and using simple techniques like inhalation and topical application, you can create a mindful, healing experience that nourishes both the body and mind.

Choosing Essential Oils for Meditation

Essential oils can significantly enhance your meditation practice by promoting relaxation, improving focus, and creating a peaceful environment. The right essential oils can help calm the mind, relieve stress, and deepen your meditation experience. When choosing essential oils for meditation, it's important to consider the specific emotional and mental effects you wish to achieve. Whether you're seeking to reduce anxiety, improve concentration, or encourage mindfulness, each essential oil offers unique benefits that can support your meditation journey.

Frankincense Oil

Frankincense is one of the most revered oils for meditation due to its deeply grounding and calming properties. Known for its ability to reduce mental chatter and enhance spiritual awareness, frankincense helps to center the mind and body, allowing for deeper states of meditation. It has a rich, resinous aroma that evokes feelings of peace and connection. Frankincense oil is often used in spiritual practices to enhance a sense of presence, making it ideal for those looking to quiet their thoughts and cultivate deeper focus.

- **Benefits**: Grounding, calming, improves focus, promotes spiritual connection.
- **Best for**: Those seeking to deepen their meditation or enhance their connection to spiritual practices.

Lavender Oil

Lavender is one of the most versatile and widely used essential oils in aromatherapy. Its calming and soothing properties make it a perfect choice for meditation, especially if you're looking to reduce stress, ease anxiety, and promote relaxation. Lavender helps quiet a racing mind, making it easier to enter a state of calm and focus. It is ideal for beginners, as it helps set a tranquil environment for meditation, allowing you to release tension and become more present.

- **Benefits**: Stress reduction, relaxation, mental clarity, emotional balance.
- **Best for**: Those new to meditation or those needing help calming anxious or restless thoughts.

Sandalwood Oil

Sandalwood oil is well-known for its deep, woody aroma, which has grounding effects that help calm the nervous system. Sandalwood promotes mental clarity and focus, making it an excellent choice for those practicing mindfulness meditation. It also supports emotional balance and fosters a meditative mindset, helping you stay present in the moment. The aroma of sandalwood has a soothing quality that enhances relaxation and facilitates a peaceful environment for meditation.

- **Benefits**: Grounding, enhances focus, promotes relaxation, emotional balance.
- **Best for**: Those looking to improve concentration and deepen their mindfulness practice.

4. Bergamot Oil

Bergamot oil, derived from the peel of the bergamot orange, is known for its uplifting and mood-enhancing properties. While it is calming, it also has the ability to alleviate feelings of sadness or tension, making it an excellent choice for uplifting your mood during meditation. Bergamot oil helps release emotional blockages, reduce anxiety, and bring a sense of peace and joy. It can help open the heart and mind, allowing you to embrace a deeper sense of acceptance and calm during meditation.

- **Benefits**: Uplifting, anxiety relief, mood-enhancing, emotional release.
- **Best for**: Those needing an emotional boost or relief from tension and anxiety.

5. Peppermint Oil

Peppermint oil is a refreshing, invigorating essential oil that stimulates the mind and clears mental fog. It is especially beneficial for improving concentration and focus during meditation, making it ideal for practices that require deep attention or mental clarity. Peppermint helps open the sinuses and improves breathing, which is essential for mindfulness meditation and breathwork. The refreshing scent can help you stay alert and focused, especially during longer meditation sessions.

- **Benefits**: Mental clarity, focus, invigorating, improves breathing.
- **Best for**: Those looking to enhance mental clarity and stay awake and alert during meditation.

6. Ylang-Ylang Oil

Ylang-ylang oil, with its sweet, floral fragrance, is known for its emotional balancing effects. It helps reduce feelings of stress and emotional overwhelm, making it an excellent choice for emotional healing during meditation. Ylang-ylang promotes relaxation and self-love, encouraging emotional release and deep inner peace. It can help quiet negative emotions and restore harmony, making it ideal for meditation focused on self-compassion or healing from emotional pain.

- **Benefits**: Emotional balance, relaxation, self-love, reduces stress.
- **Best for**: Those looking to release emotional blockages or practice self-compassion.

Cedarwood Oil

Cedarwood oil has a rich, woody scent that promotes a sense of grounding and calm. It is often used in meditation for its ability to balance the mind and promote inner strength and resilience. Cedarwood helps reduce mental distractions and promotes clarity, making it ideal for those practicing focused meditation or visualization. Its earthy aroma creates a sense of safety and stability, allowing for deeper relaxation and reflection.

- **Benefits**: Grounding, clarity, emotional stability, reduces distractions.
- **Best for**: Those looking to deepen their meditation practice or achieve emotional stability.

Patchouli Oil

Patchouli oil is known for its earthy, musky aroma, which has grounding and balancing effects. It is particularly useful for deepening meditation and connecting with the earth. Patchouli helps calm the mind, ease tension, and promote relaxation. It is an excellent choice for those practicing meditation to release negative emotions or to ground themselves in their body during mindfulness practices. Patchouli helps create a peaceful environment and enhances the meditative experience.

- **Benefits**: Grounding, relaxation, emotional release, stress relief.
- **Best for**: Those seeking to ground themselves and deepen their meditation practice.

Lemon Oil

Lemon oil is known for its refreshing and invigorating aroma, making it a great choice for meditation sessions that require mental clarity and focus. Its **antioxidant** and **antibacterial** properties help clear the mind and improve concentration, making it ideal for those seeking clarity during mindfulness or concentration-based meditation. Lemon oil's uplifting scent promotes feelings of happiness and energy, making it a great choice when you need a mental refresh during meditation.

- **Benefits**: Mental clarity, focus, uplifting, refreshing.
- **Best for**: Those needing to clear mental fog and achieve focus during meditation.

10. Rose Oil

Rose oil is often considered one of the most powerful oils for emotional healing and heart-centered meditation. Its delicate, floral scent promotes self-love, emotional release, and compassion. Rose oil helps open the heart chakra and promotes a sense of inner peace, making it an excellent choice for meditation focused on healing emotional wounds or connecting with love and compassion. Its calming properties help soothe anxiety and bring a sense of deep relaxation.

- **Benefits**: Emotional healing, self-love, compassion, calming.
- **Best for**: Those seeking emotional healing, love-based meditation, or deeper relaxation.

How to Use Essential Oils for Meditation

There are several ways to incorporate essential oils into your meditation practice:

- **Diffuser**: Use a diffuser to fill the room with the calming or uplifting aroma of your chosen essential oil, creating an atmosphere conducive to meditation.
- **Topical Application**: Dilute essential oils in a carrier oil and apply them to pulse points (temples, wrists, or the back of the neck) to support relaxation or focus.
- **Inhalation**: Simply inhale the aroma of essential oils by placing a few drops in your hands or on a cloth and breathing deeply. This can help calm the mind and prepare you for meditation.
- **Aromatherapy Roller Blends**: You can create a portable roller blend with your favorite essential oils to apply right before meditation for instant relaxation and focus.

By choosing the right essential oils and incorporating them into your meditation practice, you can deepen your connection to your inner self, enhance focus, and experience a more transformative meditation session.

Learning to Use Aromatherapy in Your Practice

Aromatherapy is a powerful and versatile tool that can enhance your personal well-being and mindfulness practice. By incorporating essential oils into your routine, you can deepen your relaxation, improve focus, reduce stress, and promote emotional balance. The beauty of aromatherapy lies in its simplicity and its ability to support various aspects of physical, emotional, and mental health, offering a holistic approach to wellness. Whether you're a beginner or experienced in using essential oils, understanding how to incorporate them into your daily life can help you harness their full potential.

Understanding Essential Oils

Essential oils are concentrated plant extracts that capture the natural healing properties of herbs, flowers, fruits, and trees. They are typically used in aromatherapy to influence the body and mind through inhalation or topical application. Each oil carries distinct benefits, such as **relaxation, mental clarity**, or **mood enhancement**, making them ideal for supporting various aspects of your well-being. Learning which essential oils align with your goals—whether for stress reduction, focus, emotional healing, or energy boost—is the first step toward creating a beneficial aromatherapy practice.

How to Use Essential Oils in Your Practice

The most common methods for using essential oils are **diffusion, topical application,** and **inhalation**. Each technique has its own unique benefits and can be tailored to your needs.

- **Diffusion**: Using an essential oil diffuser is one of the most popular ways to enjoy the benefits of aromatherapy. By dispersing essential oils into the air, a diffuser helps create a calming atmosphere, clear your mind, and improve the air quality. When practicing **mindfulness, meditation,** or simply relaxing at home, diffusing oils like **lavender, frankincense**, or **bergamot** can help promote peace and tranquility.
- **Topical Application**: Applying diluted essential oils directly to the skin allows the oils to be absorbed, benefiting your body on a deeper level. For example, **peppermint oil** can be massaged into your temples to help with headaches, or **tea tree oil** can be used on sore muscles for its anti-inflammatory properties. Always

dilute essential oils with a carrier oil, such as **jojoba, coconut,** or **sweet almond oil**, to avoid irritation and ensure safe application.
- **Inhalation**: Inhaling essential oils directly is one of the quickest ways to absorb their therapeutic properties. Simply add a few drops of your chosen oil to a handkerchief, cotton ball, or your palms, and inhale deeply. **Eucalyptus, peppermint,** and **lemon** are great oils for promoting clear breathing and stimulating alertness, while **lavender** and **chamomile** work wonders for calming the mind during times of stress.

Integrating Aromatherapy into Daily Practices

Aromatherapy can be integrated seamlessly into daily routines to enhance your overall well-being. Here are a few ways to incorporate essential oils into various aspects of your practice:

- **Morning Routine**: Start your day with energizing oils to boost your mood and prepare your mind for the day ahead. **Citrus oils** like **lemon, orange,** or **grapefruit** are uplifting and promote a sense of refreshment. **Peppermint oil** is also a great choice to invigorate the senses and provide mental clarity. Diffusing these oils while drinking your morning tea or engaging in light stretches can help center your focus.
- **Mindfulness and Meditation**: Essential oils are excellent companions for mindfulness practices, where they can enhance your ability to stay present. Use calming oils such as **lavender, frankincense,** or **sandalwood** in your meditation space to promote relaxation and grounding. Diffuse or apply the oil to pulse points like your wrists or temples to deepen your focus and create an atmosphere conducive to stillness.
- **Stress Relief**: During stressful moments, aromatherapy offers an effective way to unwind. **Lavender, chamomile,** and **ylang-ylang** are great for easing anxiety and restoring balance. Consider a calming massage with **lavender oil** and a carrier oil, or a relaxing bath with **frankincense** and **cedarwood** to melt away tension. Taking deep breaths while inhaling these oils can help calm the nervous system and provide immediate relief.
- **Sleep Support**: Essential oils can support better sleep by promoting relaxation and calm. Oils like **lavender, cedarwood,** and **vetiver** are known for their sleep-inducing qualities. You can diffuse these oils in your bedroom or apply them topically before bed to create a peaceful, restful environment. Adding a few drops to your pillow or blanket can further enhance the calming atmosphere.

Choosing the Right Essential Oils for Your Needs

When selecting essential oils, consider your individual needs and preferences. Here are some common uses for specific oils:

- **For Relaxation**: Lavender, chamomile, and ylang-ylang are excellent choices for calming the mind and promoting emotional balance.
- **For Focus**: Peppermint, rosemary, and basil are stimulating oils that can help improve concentration and mental clarity.
- **For Stress and Anxiety**: Bergamot, frankincense, and sandalwood offer grounding effects that help alleviate stress and promote emotional well-being.
- **For Energy**: Citrus oils such as lemon, orange, and grapefruit provide a refreshing, uplifting boost, perfect for boosting energy and mood.

Creating Personalized Blends

One of the most enjoyable aspects of using aromatherapy is crafting personalized blends that suit your individual preferences and needs. You can experiment by combining different oils to enhance their benefits. For example, a blend of **lavender, frankincense, and sandalwood** creates a deeply relaxing and grounding blend for meditation or evening relaxation. A combination of **peppermint, lemon,** and **rosemary** can help invigorate the mind and boost focus during work or study sessions.

Start by blending a few drops of each oil in a small glass bottle or rollerball applicator with a carrier oil. Test your blend and adjust the ratios as needed. Keep a journal of your blends so you can remember which ones worked best for specific moments or needs.

Safety Considerations

While essential oils are generally safe when used properly, it's important to follow a few safety guidelines:

- Always dilute essential oils with a carrier oil before applying them to the skin to avoid irritation.
- Perform a patch test on a small area of skin before using a new oil to ensure you don't have an allergic reaction.
- Keep essential oils out of reach of children, and avoid using certain oils during pregnancy or if you have specific health concerns.
- If you have sensitive skin or conditions such as eczema, consult with a healthcare provider before using certain oils.

Conclusion

Learning how to incorporate aromatherapy into your daily practice is a simple yet effective way to enhance your well-being. Whether you are looking to relax, improve focus, manage stress, or enhance your meditation practice, essential oils offer a natural and holistic solution. By understanding how to choose and use essential oils, you can tailor your aromatherapy practice to meet your specific needs, creating a therapeutic experience that supports both your body and mind.

Aromatherapy in Your Daily Routine

Aromatherapy is a simple yet powerful tool that can be easily incorporated into your daily routine to enhance your overall well-being. The use of essential oils, whether through inhalation, topical application, or diffusion, provides natural support for various aspects of health, from mental clarity and relaxation to improved skin health and immunity. By integrating aromatherapy into your everyday activities, you can create a calming, uplifting, and healing environment that supports both physical and emotional balance.

Morning Routine: Energizing and Uplifting

Start your day by incorporating essential oils that boost your energy, improve mood, and help you feel focused and refreshed. Citrus oils like **lemon, grapefruit**, and **orange** are perfect for a morning lift, as they are known for their **uplifting, refreshing**, and **energizing** qualities. These oils can help wake up the senses and set a positive tone for the day.

- **Diffusion**: Add a few drops of **lemon** or **grapefruit** oil to a diffuser to fill the room with an invigorating scent that boosts your mood and clears mental fog.
- **Topical Application**: Dilute **peppermint** oil with a carrier oil and apply it to your wrists or temples to invigorate your mind and promote alertness.
- **Inhalation**: You can also place a few drops of **eucalyptus** or **peppermint** oil on a cotton ball and breathe deeply as you prepare for the day. This can help clear the airways and improve focus.

During Work or Study: Enhancing Focus and Clarity

Throughout the day, especially during work or study, aromatherapy can help you stay focused, improve concentration, and reduce mental fatigue. Essential oils like **rosemary, basil**, and **peppermint** are great for boosting cognitive function, supporting memory retention, and maintaining alertness.

- **Diffusion**: Diffuse **rosemary** oil to enhance mental clarity and focus, creating a productive environment.
- **Topical Application**: Apply diluted **basil** oil or **peppermint** oil to the back of the neck or your temples to stimulate your senses and refresh your mind.

- **Inhalation**: A few deep breaths of **lemon** or **rosemary** essential oil can clear your mind and help you stay alert, especially when working on tasks that require sustained concentration.

Afternoon Slump: Recharging Your Energy

After lunch, it's common to experience a dip in energy or productivity, but a few simple aromatherapy practices can help revive your focus and energy. **Citrus oils**, like **orange** or **grapefruit**, are perfect for combating sluggishness and boosting motivation in the afternoon.

- **Diffusion**: Refresh your space with a citrusy blend of **lemon** and **bergamot** oils in a diffuser to help energize your body and mind.
- **Topical Application**: Apply a roller blend containing **peppermint** and **lemon** oil to your pulse points for a quick pick-me-up.
- **Inhalation**: Breathe deeply from a bottle or cloth infused with **eucalyptus** or **peppermint** oil to reinvigorate your senses.

Stress Relief in the Evening: Unwinding and Relaxing

Aromatherapy is particularly beneficial in the evening to promote relaxation and relieve the stress that has accumulated throughout the day. Essential oils like **lavender**, **chamomile**, and **frankincense** are ideal for helping you unwind and prepare for a restful night's sleep.

- **Diffusion**: Diffuse calming oils such as **lavender** and **frankincense** in the evening to promote relaxation and create a tranquil atmosphere in your home.
- **Topical Application**: Add a few drops of **lavender** oil to your temples, wrists, or the back of your neck to help reduce stress and promote emotional calm.
- **Inhalation**: Inhale deeply from a bottle of **chamomile** or **lavender** oil to calm your mind, relieve tension, and prepare for sleep.

Self-Care and Skincare Routine: Nourishing Your Body

Incorporating essential oils into your skincare routine is a great way to nourish and care for your skin while benefiting from their therapeutic properties. Essential oils like **tea tree**, **geranium**, and **rose** are excellent for addressing skin issues, such as acne, dry patches, and signs of aging.

- **Topical Application**: Add a few drops of **tea tree** oil to your moisturizer or acne treatment to help reduce blemishes and promote clear skin. For dry or sensitive skin, **rose** oil can be mixed into your moisturizer to hydrate and restore balance.

- **Facial Steam**: For a refreshing facial treatment, add a few drops of **lavender** or **chamomile** oil to hot water and inhale the steam to cleanse and soothe your skin.
- **Massage**: Use a blend of **geranium** and **jojoba** oil to massage your face, helping to improve circulation and promote a radiant, glowing complexion.

Nighttime Routine: Promoting Restful Sleep

Getting enough restful sleep is essential for overall well-being, and aromatherapy can support a more peaceful night's sleep. Essential oils like **lavender, cedarwood,** and **vetiver** are particularly helpful in calming the mind and encouraging deep, restorative rest.

- **Diffusion**: Diffuse **lavender** and **cedarwood** oils in your bedroom before bed to create a calming atmosphere that supports sleep. These oils help relax the mind, ease anxiety, and promote a restful environment.
- **Topical Application**: Apply diluted **lavender** oil to your pulse points or feet before bed to ease tension and promote relaxation.
- **Inhalation**: For a sleep-enhancing boost, inhale a few deep breaths of **chamomile** or **vetiver** oil just before settling into bed to relax and prepare for sleep.

Essential Oil Blends for Daily Use

Creating personalized essential oil blends can enhance your aromatherapy experience. For example, a **calming** blend for the evening could include **lavender, chamomile,** and **cedarwood**. A **focus-boosting** blend for work might combine **rosemary, peppermint,** and **lemon** oils. These blends can be used in a diffuser, diluted for topical application, or inhaled throughout the day to support your specific needs.

Conclusion

Incorporating aromatherapy into your daily routine is a simple yet powerful way to improve your physical and emotional well-being. Whether it's to energize your morning, focus during work, relieve stress, or promote better sleep, essential oils provide a natural and effective solution for enhancing your overall quality of life. By choosing oils that support your goals and integrating them into your daily practices, you can create a therapeutic, calming, and invigorating atmosphere that benefits both your body and mind.

Simple Ways to Incorporate Aromatherapy into your Life

Aromatherapy is a simple yet effective way to enhance your well-being using the therapeutic power of essential oils. Whether you're looking to reduce stress, boost your mood, or improve sleep quality, there are countless ways to incorporate aromatherapy into your daily life. You don't need complicated equipment or a lot of time—small changes can make a significant impact on your physical, emotional, and mental health.

1. Diffusing Essential Oils

One of the easiest and most common ways to incorporate aromatherapy is through diffusing essential oils into your living space. A diffuser disperses the oils into the air, creating a calming or energizing atmosphere depending on your needs.

- **For relaxation**: Use oils like **lavender, chamomile,** or **frankincense** to promote soothing environment, especially during times of stress or before bed.
- **For energy: Citrus oils** like **lemon, orange,** or **grapefruit** are invigorating and uplifting, making them ideal for mornings or when you need a mid-day energy boost.

Simply add a few drops of your chosen oil to the diffuser, fill it with water, and let the aroma fill the room. This method is particularly helpful for creating a peaceful environment while working, meditating, or winding down.

2. Aromatherapy Baths

Taking a bath infused with essential oils is an excellent way to relax your muscles, hydrate your skin, and soothe your mind. Adding a few drops of essential oils to your bathwater allows you to enjoy their benefits while bathing.

- **For relaxation and sleep: Lavender** and **cedarwood** oils help calm the mind and prepare the body for restful sleep.
- **For muscle relief: Eucalyptus** and **peppermint** oils are ideal for alleviating sore muscles and clearing your sinuses.

mix the oils with a carrier oil (like coconut or olive oil) to ensure they disperse evenly in the water, as essential oils are not water-soluble. Soaking in an aromatherapy bath can become a soothing ritual, especially at the end of a stressful day.

Essential Oil Massage

Incorporating essential oils into your massage routine is a fantastic way to relax your body and relieve tension. Massage not only works the muscles but can also promote the absorption of essential oils through the skin, allowing their therapeutic properties to take effect.

- **For muscle relaxation**: **Peppermint**, **rosemary**, or **lavender** oils help ease tension and alleviate sore muscles.
- **For stress relief**: A calming blend of **chamomile, lavender,** and **sandalwood** oils can help relax both the body and mind.

Dilute essential oils with a carrier oil (such as jojoba or almond oil) and use gentle strokes to apply the blend to areas that need attention. A self-massage with your favorite aromatherapy oils can help you wind down after a long day.

Inhalation and Personal Aromatherapy

Inhaling essential oils directly is one of the quickest and most effective ways to enjoy their benefits. This can be done through various methods, such as applying oils to a cotton ball, inhaling from a bottle, or using an aromatherapy inhaler.

- **For mental clarity and focus**: **Peppermint**, **rosemary**, and **lemon** oils can help clear your mind and improve concentration, making them perfect for work or study.
- **For relaxation and anxiety relief**: Inhale deeply from a bottle of **lavender** or **frankincense** oil to calm your nerves and reduce stress.

You can also carry an essential oil roller with you throughout the day for a quick inhalation boost whenever needed.

Aromatherapy Skincare

Incorporating essential oils into your skincare routine can enhance the effects of your existing products, offering both physical and emotional benefits. Adding a few drops of essential oils to your moisturizer, face mask, or body lotion can provide targeted skin care and promote relaxation.

- **For glowing skin**: **Tea tree** oil is great for acne-prone skin, while **rose** oil hydrates and revitalizes dry skin.
- **For soothing irritated skin**: **Chamomile** and **lavender** oils can help reduce inflammation and calm skin conditions like eczema or redness.

Make sure to dilute the oils in a carrier oil before applying them to your skin to prevent irritation, especially on the face or sensitive areas.

6. Aromatherapy on the Go

Aromatherapy doesn't have to be confined to your home—essential oils can be part of your routine even when you're out and about. Essential oil rollers, which are small and portable, can be used to bring a dose of relaxation or energy wherever you go.

- **For stress relief during busy days**: Carry a roller with **lavender** or **bergamot** for a calming effect during work or social events.
- **For boosting energy**: A roller with **peppermint** or **citrus oils** can help reinvigorate you during moments of fatigue.

Simply roll the essential oils onto your pulse points (wrists, neck, or temples) for a quick and easy aromatherapy experience on the go.

7. Cleaning and Purifying the Home

Essential oils can also be used for more practical purposes, such as cleaning and purifying the air in your home. Many essential oils, like **tea tree**, **eucalyptus**, and **lemon** have **antibacterial**, **antiviral**, and **antifungal** properties that can help cleanse your living space.

- **For a fresh, clean scent**: Use a blend of **lemon**, **rosemary**, and **peppermint** oil to create a natural and refreshing cleaning solution for your home.
- **For purifying the air**: Diffuse **eucalyptus**, **lavender**, or **tea tree** oil to eliminate odors, refresh the atmosphere, and promote better air quality.

Essential oils make a great addition to natural cleaning routines, offering both effective cleaning power and a pleasing aroma.

8. Meditation and Mindfulness

Aromatherapy is an excellent complement to meditation and mindfulness practices. By diffusing calming essential oils, you can create a peaceful space that enhances your ability to focus, relax, and connect with your inner self.

- **For grounding**: **Sandalwood** and **cedarwood** oils are perfect for centering yourself during meditation, promoting a deeper sense of presence.
- **For relaxation**: **Lavender**, **frankincense**, and **chamomile** oils help quiet the mind and reduce distractions, aiding in deeper relaxation and mindfulness.

Incorporating essential oils into your meditation practice can elevate your experience and help you achieve a more profound state of calm and clarity.

Conclusion

Incorporating aromatherapy into your daily routine is a simple yet effective way to improve both physical and emotional well-being. Whether through diffusion, topical application, skincare, or meditation, essential oils offer a natural way to reduce stress, enhance focus, and improve mood. With just a few drops of your favorite oils, you can transform your home, workplace, and personal care regimen into a holistic wellness experience that promotes balance, relaxation, and vitality throughout your day.

Making Your Own Aromatherapy Products

Creating your own aromatherapy products is a rewarding way to bring the therapeutic benefits of essential oils into your daily life. Whether you're making a relaxing massage oil, a refreshing body spray, or a soothing bath salt blend, the process allows you to customize products to suit your personal needs, preferences, and wellness goals. With just a few basic ingredients and some essential oils, you can craft high-quality, natural products that promote relaxation, health, and overall well-being.

1. Aromatherapy Massage Oil

Massage oils infused with essential oils are perfect for soothing sore muscles, reducing tension, and enhancing relaxation. The process of massaging the oil into your skin helps the essential oils penetrate more deeply, while the act itself is beneficial for stress relief and improving circulation.

Ingredients:

- 1/4 cup of **carrier oil** (such as **jojoba**, **sweet almond**, or **coconut oil**)
- 10-15 drops of your preferred essential oil(s) (such as **lavender** for relaxation, **peppermint** for muscle relief, or **rosemary** for circulation)

Instructions:

1. In a small glass bottle, mix the carrier oil with your essential oils.
2. Shake well to combine.
3. Use as needed for a relaxing massage, applying the oil to areas of tension or discomfort.

Tip: If you want to create a specific blend for different purposes, try combining oils like **lavender** and **chamomile** for relaxation or **peppermint** and **eucalyptus** for muscle soreness and improved breathing.

2. Aromatherapy Body Scrub

An aromatherapy body scrub exfoliates the skin while offering the benefits of essential oils. It removes dead skin cells, leaving your skin feeling soft and smooth, and the essential oils can provide an added boost to your wellness routine, such as relaxation or invigoration.

Ingredients:

- 1/2 cup of **sugar** (or **sea salt** for a more intense scrub)
- 1/4 cup of **carrier oil** (like **coconut oil** or **olive oil**)
- 10-15 drops of essential oils (such as **orange** and **eucalyptus** for an energizing scrub or **lavender** and **chamomile** for a calming effect)

Instructions:

1. In a bowl, mix the sugar or salt with the carrier oil until you achieve a paste-like consistency.
2. Add the essential oils and stir until evenly distributed.
3. Store in an airtight container and use in the shower, gently scrubbing your body in circular motions.

Tip: If you want to target specific skin concerns, such as dryness, you can add a tablespoon of **honey** for extra moisture, or for extra relaxation, try adding a few drops of **frankincense** or **rose** oil.

Aromatherapy Bath Salts

Aromatherapy bath salts are an excellent way to unwind after a long day, with the added benefits of both aromatherapy and skin nourishment. The minerals in Epsom salt can help relax muscles, while essential oils offer a calming or rejuvenating atmosphere.

Ingredients:

- 1 cup of **Epsom salts**
- 1/2 cup of **sea salt**
- 10-15 drops of essential oils (for relaxation, try **lavender**, **chamomile**, or **sandalwood**)

Instructions:

1. In a mixing bowl, combine the Epsom salt and sea salt.
2. Add the essential oils and stir thoroughly to ensure the oils are evenly distributed.
3. Store the salts in a glass jar and use about 1/4 cup of the mix per bath. Simply add the bath salts to warm water and soak for 20-30 minutes.

Tip: For added benefits, add a tablespoon of **baking soda** to the mix to help neutralize odors and soften the skin.

4. Aromatherapy Room Spray

Room sprays are a great way to refresh your living space and create a soothing atmosphere. They can be used to neutralize odors, calm the mind, or energize the environment, depending on the essential oils you choose.

Ingredients:

- 1 cup of **distilled water**
- 2 tablespoons of **witch hazel** or **vodka** (helps the oils blend with water)
- 10-20 drops of essential oils (for relaxation, use **lavender** or **frankincense**; for a fresh, uplifting scent, try **lemon** or **peppermint**)

Instructions:

1. Combine the water, witch hazel or vodka, and essential oils in a spray bottle.
2. Shake well before each use to mix the oils and water.
3. Spray the mist around your home, in the bathroom, or on linens for a refreshing scent.

Tip: If you're using a room spray for sleep, opt for **lavender** and **chamomile** oils. For an energy boost or to create an inviting atmosphere, **grapefruit** and **bergamot** are great choices.

5. Aromatherapy Facial Mist

An aromatherapy facial mist is an excellent way to hydrate and refresh your skin throughout the day while benefiting from the calming effects of essential oils. It's especially useful for a quick pick-me-up or during dry seasons to maintain skin hydration.

Ingredients:

- 1/2 cup of **rose water** or **distilled water**
- 10-15 drops of essential oils (try **lavender** for calming, **geranium** for balancing, or **rose** for hydration)

Instructions:

1. Mix the rose water or distilled water with the essential oils in a spray bottle.
2. Shake well before each use.
3. Spray lightly over your face, holding the bottle about 8-10 inches away.

p: For a cooling effect in warmer weather, add a few drops of **peppermint** oil to your st. If you have sensitive skin, be sure to patch-test the mist before full application.

Aromatherapy Candles

aking your own aromatherapy candles is a fun and creative way to enjoy the benefits of sential oils. Candles provide not only light and warmth but also release a subtle aroma o your environment, enhancing the mood of any room.

gredients:

- **Soy wax** (or beeswax) for a clean burn
- 10-15 drops of essential oils (use **lavender** for relaxation, **citrus oils** for energy, or **sandalwood** for grounding)
- A candle wick and container (such as a mason jar or glass votive)

structions:

1. Melt the wax according to the package instructions (usually in a double boiler).
2. Once melted, add the essential oils to the wax and stir.
3. Pour the mixture into your container, securing the wick in the center.
4. Allow the candle to cool and harden completely before lighting.

p: Experiment with different combinations of oils to create your own signature scent, choose oils that align with the season (e.g., **cinnamon** and **clove** for autumn).

onclusion

aking your own aromatherapy products is a creative and personalized way to integrate e power of essential oils into your daily life. Whether you are crafting a calming assage oil, an energizing room spray, or a relaxing bath soak, the possibilities are dless. By using natural ingredients and high-quality essential oils, you can create oducts that cater to your specific needs and preferences, all while embracing the erapeutic benefits of aromatherapy.

Exploring Advanced Aromatherapy Techniques

Aromatherapy is a versatile practice that can be tailored to address a wide variety of physical and emotional concerns. While basic methods like diffusion and topical application are commonly used, there are more advanced techniques that can deepen the therapeutic effects of essential oils. These techniques enhance the efficacy of aromatherapy, addressing specific health concerns or intensifying the experience of relaxation, healing, and mental clarity.

1. Aromatherapy Inhalation Techniques

Inhalation is one of the quickest ways for essential oils to reach the brain, particularly the limbic system, which governs emotions, memory, and behavior. While simple inhalation can be done by breathing directly from a bottle or diffuser, advanced inhalation techniques can be more intentional and focused.

- **Steam Inhalation**: This technique involves adding a few drops of essential oil to a bowl of hot water and inhaling the steam deeply. It's particularly beneficial for respiratory conditions like congestion, sinusitis, or even emotional overwhelm. Oils like **eucalyptus, peppermint,** and **rosemary** are excellent for clearing airways, while oils like **lavender** and **chamomile** can help calm the mind.
- **Aromatherapy Inhalers**: These portable devices allow you to inhale concentrated essential oils directly, offering a targeted method for relieving stress, boosting focus, or uplifting mood. Inhalers are particularly useful for **on-the-go aromatherapy**, as you can easily carry them in your bag for quick relief during stressful moments or to stay focused during work.

2. Aromatherapy for Chakra Balancing

Chakra balancing is a technique used in aromatherapy to help align the energy centers of the body. Each of the seven chakras corresponds to specific physical, emotional, and spiritual aspects, and the right essential oils can help restore balance to these areas.

- **Root Chakra**: To ground and stabilize energy, **cedarwood, vetiver,** and **patchouli** are used for their earthy, calming properties. These oils help provide a sense of security and connection to the Earth.

- **Heart Chakra**: To encourage love and compassion, oils like **rose**, **ylang-ylang**, and **geranium** are applied. These oils support emotional healing, forgiveness, and open-heartedness.
- **Third Eye Chakra**: **Frankincense**, **lavender**, and **sandalwood** are commonly used to stimulate intuition, awareness, and insight. These oils can help clear mental fog and enhance spiritual connection.

To perform a chakra balancing treatment, you can diffuse the oils or apply them directly to the skin, focusing on the corresponding chakra points (i.e., the base of the spine, heart area, forehead). Meditation or focused breathing can also be incorporated to enhance the benefits of the oils.

Aromatherapy for Energy Healing and Emotional Detox

Aromatherapy can be an effective tool for emotional healing by using essential oils to facilitate the release of negative emotions and energy blockages. Advanced techniques involve more intentional methods of emotional clearing, helping to break through emotional stagnation and promote healing.

- **Emotional Release with Essential Oils**: Certain oils, such as **frankincense**, **rose**, and **sandalwood**, are believed to help release deep-seated emotions like grief, anger, or fear. These oils support emotional clarity and openness. One method is to inhale these oils deeply while focusing on emotional release during meditation or journaling.
- **Energy Healing Practices**: Aromatherapy can complement energy healing practices like Reiki or acupuncture. Essential oils can be applied to energy points on the body (known as meridians) or placed in the surrounding area to enhance the flow of **chi** (energy) during treatment. Oils like **lavender** and **cedarwood** are often used to balance and stabilize the energy field, while **lemon** and **peppermint** are used for clearing and refreshing energy.

Aromatherapy Massage for Deeper Therapeutic Benefits

Advanced aromatherapy massage techniques involve not just the use of essential oils, but the application of focused pressure and movement to release muscle tension, stimulate circulation, and promote deep relaxation.

- **Acupressure with Essential Oils**: Acupressure can be enhanced by applying essential oils to specific pressure points on the body. **Peppermint** and **eucalyptus** oils are commonly used in acupressure sessions to help relieve tension and promote circulation, while **lavender** or **chamomile** is applied to induce relaxation. By massaging these oils into the acupressure points, you can deepen the effects of the treatment.

- **Lymphatic Drainage Massage**: This technique promotes the removal of toxins and waste from the body and improves immune function. **Grapefruit**, **lemon**, and **juniper berry** oils are ideal for supporting lymphatic health. These oils can be blended with a carrier oil and used in long, sweeping strokes along the lymphatic pathways to encourage detoxification and relieve stagnation.

5. Aromatherapy for Sleep Enhancement

For those struggling with insomnia or poor sleep quality, advanced aromatherapy techniques can help promote restful, uninterrupted sleep by calming the nervous system and soothing the mind.

- **Sleep Inducing Diffusion**: While basic diffusing of sleep-inducing oils like **lavender, chamomile**, and **bergamot** can be effective, advanced methods involve blending multiple oils that synergistically support relaxation and sleep. A calming blend of **lavender, cedarwood**, and **vetiver** can be used in a diffuser or applied topically to the feet and pulse points for deep sleep.
- **Aromatherapy Sleep Mask**: To enhance sleep during the night, you can apply a few drops of **lavender** or **frankincense** to a sleep mask. This allows you to breathe in the oils during sleep, promoting a restful environment even while you're unconscious.

6. Advanced Aromatherapy for Skin Care

Aromatherapy can also play a crucial role in advanced skincare techniques, particularly for those dealing with specific skin conditions, signs of aging, or overall skin health.

- **Anti-Aging and Skin Repair**: Essential oils such as **rose, frankincense**, and **helichrysum** are known for their regenerative and rejuvenating properties. These oils help stimulate cell regeneration, reduce the appearance of fine lines, and promote skin elasticity. By incorporating these oils into a serum or facial cream, you can create a potent anti-aging treatment.
- **Healing Scars and Skin Imperfections**: **Lavender** and **tea tree oil** are effective for treating acne and promoting skin healing. **Helichrysum** oil is particularly useful for scar healing, as it helps to regenerate tissue and reduce the appearance of scars or stretch marks. Applying diluted oils directly to the affected areas or using them in a massage oil blend can enhance the skin's natural healing processes.

7. Aromatherapy for Manifestation and Intent Setting

Aromatherapy can also support your spiritual practice by enhancing the process of manifestation and intention setting. The oils you choose can align with specific desires or goals, helping to manifest them into your life.

- **Essential Oils for Manifestation**: **Jasmine**, **rose**, and **frankincense** are commonly used in manifestation rituals to amplify energy and open the heart. These oils are believed to enhance creativity, attraction, and abundance. During meditation or intention-setting rituals, you can use these oils to focus on the positive energy you want to bring into your life.
- **Affirmations with Essential Oils**: Pairing essential oils with affirmations can help you stay aligned with your intentions. For example, while diffusing **bergamot** or **cedarwood**, you could affirm statements like, "I am grounded and focused" or "I attract positive energy into my life."

Conclusion

By exploring advanced aromatherapy techniques, you can deepen your connection to both your physical and emotional health. Whether you're using essential oils for emotional healing, skin care, enhanced meditation, or muscle relief, the possibilities for using aromatherapy are vast. Through mindful application and intention, you can unlock the full potential of essential oils and bring profound therapeutic benefits into your life.

Understanding the Chakras and Aromatherapy

Chakras are energy centers within the body that correspond to different physical, emotional, and spiritual aspects of well-being. According to traditional Indian medicine and yoga philosophy, there are seven primary chakras that align along the spine, each associated with specific functions and emotional states. Aromatherapy can play a powerful role in balancing and healing these chakras, as essential oils have the ability to influence both the physical body and the subtle energy systems. By understanding the chakras and how specific essential oils can support them, you can enhance your physical health, emotional resilience, and spiritual growth.

Root Chakra (Muladhara)

The Root Chakra is located at the base of the spine and is associated with feelings of stability, security, and grounding. When balanced, this chakra promotes a sense of physical health, safety, and connection to the Earth. An imbalanced root chakra can lead to feelings of fear, insecurity, or financial instability.

- **Essential Oils for Root Chakra**: To ground and stabilize energy, **cedarwood**, **patchouli**, and **vetiver** are ideal. These oils have earthy, grounding properties that help reconnect you to the Earth and strengthen your sense of security. **Frankincense** and **myrrh** also promote grounding, clarity, and strength, making them excellent choices for supporting the root chakra.

Usage: Diffuse these oils in your space, or apply them diluted with a carrier oil to the base of your spine, feet, or ankles to help ground yourself during meditation or stressful situations.

Sacral Chakra (Svadhisthana)

The Sacral Chakra is located in the lower abdomen, near the reproductive organs, and is associated with creativity, passion, and emotional expression. This chakra governs your ability to form relationships and experience pleasure. When blocked or unbalanced, it can manifest as creative blockages, emotional instability, or difficulties in intimacy.

- **Essential Oils for Sacral Chakra**: Oils like **sweet orange, ylang-ylang, jasmine**, and **geranium** can help activate and balance this chakra. These oils are known for their uplifting, sensual, and emotionally opening properties, which help release blockages and encourage creativity and emotional flow.

Usage: Apply diluted oils to the lower abdomen or use them in a diffuser during creative practices, emotional work, or relaxation exercises to foster emotional freedom and vitality.

Solar Plexus Chakra (Manipura)

The Solar Plexus Chakra, located in the upper abdomen around the stomach, is the center of personal power, self-esteem, and confidence. When balanced, it supports your ability to make decisions, assert yourself, and take control of your life. An imbalanced solar plexus chakra can lead to feelings of inadequacy, low energy, or difficulty asserting boundaries.

- **Essential Oils for Solar Plexus Chakra**: **Lemon, ginger, peppermint**, and **rosemary** are great choices for stimulating the solar plexus. These oils have invigorating and energizing properties that help clear mental fog, boost confidence, and enhance personal power. **Bergamot** can also help alleviate anxiety and foster emotional balance.

Usage: To activate the solar plexus chakra, apply essential oils diluted in a carrier oil to the upper abdomen or solar plexus area, or diffuse them in your space to uplift your energy and self-confidence.

Heart Chakra (Anahata)

The Heart Chakra is located in the center of the chest and governs love, compassion, and emotional balance. It serves as the bridge between the physical and spiritual realms. A balanced heart chakra promotes kindness, empathy, and deep connections with others. When unbalanced, it can manifest as feelings of grief, loneliness, or difficulty forming meaningful relationships.

- **Essential Oils for Heart Chakra**: **Rose, geranium, lavender**, and **chamomile** are known for their heart-opening and calming properties. These oils help promote emotional healing, compassion, and self-love. **Bergamot** and **ylang-ylang** also encourage a balanced emotional state and help alleviate feelings of sadness or emotional blockages.

Usage: Apply diluted oils to the chest area or diffuse them to enhance emotional healing, promote love and compassion, and foster a deeper connection to yourself and others.

Throat Chakra (Vishuddha)

The Throat Chakra is located at the throat and is responsible for communication, self-expression, and speaking your truth. It governs how you express your thoughts and feelings, both verbally and non-verbally. When this chakra is balanced, it allows for clear, honest communication. An imbalanced throat chakra can lead to fear of speaking, difficulty expressing yourself, or physical issues like sore throats.

- **Essential Oils for Throat Chakra**: **Peppermint**, **eucalyptus**, **lavender**, and **chamomile** are excellent oils for opening the throat chakra. These oils help clear blockages in communication and promote clarity of thought and speech. **Clary sage** and **frankincense** also support the expression of truth and creativity.

Usage: Apply diluted oils to the throat or diffuse them during meditation, journaling, or public speaking. These oils help release emotional blockages and promote authentic self-expression.

Third Eye Chakra (Ajna)

The Third Eye Chakra is located in the forehead, between the eyebrows, and is associated with intuition, wisdom, and mental clarity. This chakra governs your ability to perceive beyond the physical world and access your inner wisdom. When balanced, it enhances your intuition and ability to see the bigger picture. An imbalanced third eye chakra can lead to confusion, lack of direction, or difficulty trusting your instincts.

- **Essential Oils for Third Eye Chakra**: **Frankincense**, **sandalwood**, **clary sage**, and **lavender** are ideal for stimulating the third eye. These oils help promote mental clarity, intuition, and spiritual awareness. **Peppermint** and **rosemary** also support focus and clear thinking.

Usage: Apply diluted oils to the forehead, between the eyebrows, or diffuse them during meditation or mindfulness practices to enhance your intuitive abilities and clear mental blockages.

Crown Chakra (Sahasrara)

The Crown Chakra is located at the top of the head and is associated with spiritual connection, higher consciousness, and enlightenment. It governs your connection to the divine, the universe, and your higher self. A balanced crown chakra supports feelings of peace, unity, and oneness. An imbalanced crown chakra can manifest as spiritual confusion, disconnection, or a lack of purpose.

- **Essential Oils for Crown Chakra**: **Lavender, frankincense, rose**, and **myrrh** are excellent choices for balancing the crown chakra. These oils help promote spiritual awareness, clarity, and connection to higher consciousness. **Sandalwood** and **neroli** are also used to foster a deeper connection to the divine.

Usage: Apply diluted oils to the crown of the head or diffuse them in your space while meditating or practicing yoga to open your mind to higher awareness and deepen your spiritual practice.

Conclusion

Using aromatherapy in conjunction with chakra balancing can help harmonize your physical, emotional, and spiritual well-being. By selecting essential oils that correspond to each chakra, you can enhance your meditation, promote emotional healing, and support overall health. Whether used in a diffuser, applied topically, or integrated into your daily wellness routine, essential oils offer a natural and effective way to maintain the balance of your energy centers and achieve a sense of equilibrium and vitality.

Aromatherapy Reflexology

Aromatherapy reflexology combines the principles of two powerful therapeutic practices: aromatherapy, which uses essential oils for healing, and reflexology, a form of foot, hand, or ear massage that targets specific pressure points to promote overall health. This holistic treatment is designed to stimulate the body's natural healing processes by applying pressure to reflex points on the feet, hands, or ears while simultaneously using essential oils to enhance the therapeutic effects. The result is a deeply relaxing and rejuvenating experience that benefits both the body and mind.

How Aromatherapy Reflexology Works

Reflexology is based on the idea that certain areas on the feet, hands, and ears correspond to organs, systems, and glands throughout the body. By applying pressure to these reflex points, reflexologists aim to restore balance, improve circulation, and encourage the body to heal itself. Aromatherapy enhances this treatment by introducing essential oils, which can be absorbed through the skin and inhaled, amplifying the reflexology benefits.

The essential oils used in aromatherapy reflexology are chosen based on their therapeutic properties, such as calming, energizing, or detoxifying effects. These oils are typically diluted in a carrier oil (like **jojoba** or **coconut oil**) to ensure they are safe for topical application and can easily glide over the skin.

Choosing the Right Essential Oils for Reflexology

The essential oils selected for aromatherapy reflexology are tailored to the individual's specific needs. Some oils are chosen for their ability to relax and calm, while others are selected to invigorate, improve circulation, or aid in detoxification. Here are some commonly used oils and their benefits in reflexology:

- **Lavender**: Known for its calming and relaxing properties, **lavender** oil is frequently used in reflexology to reduce stress and anxiety, promote relaxation, and encourage restful sleep. It is particularly effective when working on the **solar plexus** and **heart reflexes**, helping to soothe emotional tension.
- **Peppermint**: Peppermint oil is invigorating and energizing, making it ideal for improving circulation, clearing sinuses, and providing a refreshing boost. It is often used when working on the **head**, **sinus**, or **digestive reflex points** to relieve tension headaches, boost mental clarity, and aid in digestive health.

- **Frankincense**: This oil is grounding and calming, making it useful for promoting deep relaxation and reducing emotional stress. **Frankincense** can be used when working on the **crown chakra** or reflex points related to the **nervous system** to enhance mindfulness and alleviate stress.
- **Eucalyptus**: Eucalyptus oil is known for its decongestant and respiratory benefits. It helps clear the airways, making it a great option for reflexology work focused on the **lungs** and **sinuses**. It can also promote relaxation and boost immunity, making it beneficial for those dealing with colds or respiratory issues.
- **Ginger**: Ginger oil has warming and stimulating properties that can help improve circulation, relieve pain, and promote digestion. It is commonly used in reflexology to target **digestive reflexes**, especially when dealing with nausea, indigestion, or bloating.

Techniques Used in Aromatherapy Reflexology

When practicing aromatherapy reflexology, the therapist will typically combine pressure point techniques with the application of essential oils. There are several techniques used in reflexology to stimulate the reflex points, each of which can be enhanced with aromatherapy oils.

- **Thumb Walking**: This technique involves using the thumb to apply pressure to specific reflex points, walking along the reflex zones to stimulate energy flow. **Lavender** or **chamomile** oils can be used to relax the client and promote a calming effect while pressure is applied to these points.
- **Finger Rotation**: The therapist uses their fingers to rotate over specific reflex points, often in circular motions. **Peppermint** or **eucalyptus** oils can be applied during this technique to invigorate the body, particularly for reflexes related to the **respiratory system** or **muscle tension**.
- **Finger and Thumb Pinching**: Pinching between the thumb and fingers targets specific reflex points that may be tight or congested. Essential oils like **frankincense** or **ginger** are often used to reduce inflammation and encourage detoxification while applying this technique.
- **Pressing and Holding**: This technique involves applying firm, sustained pressure to reflex points, typically used for deeper tissue work or to address specific issues such as muscle pain or digestive problems. **Ginger** and **rosemary** oils are commonly used in this method to relieve pain and improve circulation.

Benefits of Aromatherapy Reflexology

Combining aromatherapy and reflexology offers a wide range of benefits for both physical and mental health:

- **Stress and Anxiety Relief**: The calming properties of essential oils like **lavender** and **chamomile**, combined with the relaxing effects of reflexology, can significantly reduce stress and anxiety, promoting a sense of tranquility and relaxation.
- **Improved Circulation**: Essential oils like **peppermint** and **rosemary** can stimulate blood flow, while reflexology targets specific reflex points to enhance overall circulation. This combination can improve oxygen delivery to the body's tissues and help reduce swelling and stiffness.
- **Pain Relief**: Reflexology, paired with oils like **peppermint** and **ginger**, can help relieve muscle tension, headaches, and joint pain. The oils' anti-inflammatory properties work synergistically with the pressure techniques to ease discomfort and promote healing.
- **Digestive Health**: Reflexology can support the digestive system by targeting specific points on the feet related to digestion. Essential oils like **ginger** and **lemon** can enhance this effect by stimulating digestive function and reducing bloating or indigestion.
- **Emotional Healing**: Reflexology can help release emotional blockages, especially when combined with oils like **frankincense** or **rose**. The use of essential oils in this context promotes emotional balance, reducing feelings of sadness, grief, or frustration, and fostering a sense of emotional well-being.

DIY Aromatherapy Reflexology

If you want to experience aromatherapy reflexology at home, here's how you can incorporate both elements into a self-care routine:

1. **Foot Soak**: Begin by soaking your feet in warm water with a few drops of **lavender** or **peppermint** essential oil mixed in a carrier oil or Epsom salt. Soaking your feet before starting reflexology can help relax muscles and soften the skin, making it easier to apply pressure.
2. **Self-Reflexology**: Apply a few drops of essential oil, diluted in a carrier oil, to your feet or hands. Use your thumb or fingers to gently massage or apply pressure to the reflex points corresponding to areas that need attention. Focus on areas like the **solar plexus** for emotional release, or the **digestive points** if you're experiencing discomfort.
3. **Aromatherapy Foot Cream**: After reflexology, apply a soothing foot cream or lotion infused with **eucalyptus** or **chamomile** essential oils to nourish your feet and extend the benefits of the treatment.

Conclusion

Aromatherapy reflexology is a deeply holistic practice that combines the physical benefits of reflexology with the therapeutic effects of essential oils. By targeting specific essure points on the body and using essential oils tailored to your needs, you can perience enhanced relaxation, pain relief, emotional healing, and improved overall alth. Whether you're seeking stress relief, better circulation, or emotional balance, this egrated approach provides a powerful tool for promoting well-being.

Expanding Your Aromatherapy Knowledge

Aromatherapy is a vast and diverse field that offers a wide array of benefits for both physical and emotional well-being. As you begin to explore this holistic practice, expanding your knowledge can deepen your understanding and enhance your ability to use essential oils effectively. Whether you're a beginner or an experienced practitioner, learning about the different aspects of aromatherapy can empower you to tailor treatments to your personal needs and goals.

Understanding Essential Oils

The cornerstone of aromatherapy is the use of essential oils—highly concentrated plant extracts that capture the natural fragrance and therapeutic properties of plants. Essential oils can be derived from various plant parts, including flowers, leaves, bark, stems, and roots. Each essential oil has its unique chemical composition and healing qualities. For example, **lavender** oil is known for its calming and relaxing effects, while **peppermint** oil is often used to invigorate and stimulate the mind.

To expand your knowledge, take the time to familiarize yourself with different oils and their uses. A few key categories include:

- **Relaxing and Calming**: Lavender, chamomile, sandalwood, frankincense
- **Energizing and Uplifting**: Citrus oils like lemon, orange, and grapefruit, as well as peppermint
- **Healing and Restorative**: Tea tree oil (antimicrobial), eucalyptus (respiratory support), and rosemary (mental clarity)
- **Skin Care**: Rose, geranium, tea tree, and lavender for various skin concerns, including acne, dryness, and irritation

Learning About Aromatherapy Methods

There are several methods for using essential oils in aromatherapy, each with its unique benefits. Understanding these methods can help you choose the best approach for your health and wellness goals.

- **Diffusion**: Using an essential oil diffuser is one of the most popular ways to introduce essential oils into your environment. The oils are dispersed into the air, allowing you to inhale their benefits, which can promote relaxation, mental clarity, or mood enhancement. Diffusing essential oils in your home or office can create an uplifting atmosphere or a calming sanctuary depending on your needs.
- **Topical Application**: When applying essential oils to the skin, it is essential to dilute them with a carrier oil, such as jojoba, sweet almond, or coconut oil, to avoid irritation. This method is effective for targeting specific areas of the body, such as sore muscles, headaches, or skin conditions. Commonly used for massage, skincare, and pain relief, topical application offers direct therapeutic effects.
- **Inhalation**: Inhaling essential oils directly can provide immediate relief, especially for conditions like stress, anxiety, or respiratory issues. You can inhale oils from a tissue, cotton ball, or an inhaler, or place a few drops in a bowl of hot water and breathe in the steam. This method quickly absorbs oils into the respiratory system, providing fast relief.
- **Bathing**: Adding essential oils to your bath can enhance relaxation and offer therapeutic benefits. Oils like lavender and chamomile are often used to calm the mind and soothe the body, while peppermint or eucalyptus can stimulate and invigorate. Always dilute oils in a carrier oil or Epsom salt to ensure even distribution in the water.

Expanding Your Knowledge Through Blending

One of the most exciting aspects of aromatherapy is creating your own blends. Mixing different essential oils can target multiple issues simultaneously and create unique, personalized scents. To effectively blend oils, it's essential to understand their properties and how they interact. Generally, essential oils fall into three categories based on their volatility:

- **Top Notes**: These oils are light, fresh, and evaporate quickly. Examples include **citrus oils** like lemon, orange, and grapefruit.
- **Middle Notes**: Known as the "heart" of a blend, these oils provide depth and balance. Examples include **lavender, geranium**, and **rose**.
- **Base Notes**: These oils are heavier, more grounding, and evaporate slowly. Examples include **cedarwood, sandalwood**, and **vetiver**.

When blending oils, aim for a balance of top, middle, and base notes to create a harmonious and lasting fragrance. For instance, a calming blend for relaxation might combine **lavender** (middle note), **chamomile** (middle note), and **sandalwood** (base note). Experiment with different combinations to find what works best for you.

Understanding Safety Guidelines

While essential oils are natural, they are potent and should be used with care. Expanding your knowledge of safety guidelines will ensure that you are using aromatherapy in a safe and effective way.

- **Dilution**: Always dilute essential oils with a carrier oil before applying them to the skin. A common dilution ratio is 2-3 drops of essential oil per teaspoon of carrier oil. For children, elderly individuals, and those with sensitive skin, use even less.
- **Patch Test**: Before using a new essential oil, conduct a patch test by applying a small diluted amount to a discreet area of your skin to ensure there is no allergic reaction.
- **Avoiding Eye Contact**: Be cautious when using essential oils around the eyes and mucous membranes, as they can be irritating. If essential oils come into contact with the eyes, flush with a carrier oil, not water.
- **Consulting Professionals**: If you are pregnant, nursing, or have any medical conditions, it's a good idea to consult with a healthcare provider or a certified aromatherapist before using essential oils.

Advanced Aromatherapy Practices

As you continue to expand your knowledge, you may want to explore more advanced techniques within aromatherapy, such as **aromatherapy massage**, **chakra healing**, and **energy work**. These practices involve using essential oils to support emotional and spiritual well-being, as well as physical health.

- **Aromatherapy Massage**: Combining aromatherapy with massage therapy enhances relaxation, improves circulation, and alleviates muscle pain. The gentle pressure of massage works synergistically with the healing properties of essential oils.
- **Chakra Healing**: Essential oils are used in chakra healing to balance the body's energy centers. Specific oils, such as **frankincense** for the crown chakra or **rose** for the heart chakra, can support emotional and spiritual healing.
- **Aromatherapy for Emotional Healing**: Many advanced practitioners use essential oils to address emotional issues like anxiety, grief, or anger. Oils like **bergamot, ylang-ylang**, and **geranium** are often used in emotional healing practices to release blockages and encourage balance.

Education and Resources

To deepen your understanding of aromatherapy, consider exploring a variety of educational resources. Books, online courses, and workshops offer valuable insights into the practice, helping you gain a better understanding of essential oils, blending techniques, and safety protocols. Joining a community of aromatherapy enthusiasts or seeking guidance from certified aromatherapists can also provide support as you expand your knowledge.

Conclusion

Expanding your aromatherapy knowledge is an exciting and rewarding journey. As you explore different essential oils, blending techniques, and advanced practices, you'll unlock a wealth of benefits for your physical, emotional, and spiritual well-being. Whether you're seeking relaxation, pain relief, or emotional healing, aromatherapy offers a natural and effective way to enhance your life. With continued learning and exploration, you can harness the full potential of aromatherapy to improve your overall health and wellness.

Resources for Continuous Learning

For those eager to deepen their understanding of aromatherapy, numerous resources are available to support continuous learning. Whether you're just starting your journey or looking to advance your skills, there are a wide variety of educational tools and communities that can help you explore new aspects of essential oils, blending techniques, and the therapeutic uses of aromatherapy.

Books

Books are one of the most comprehensive ways to learn about aromatherapy, offering in-depth insights into essential oils, safety guidelines, and practical applications. Some recommended titles include:

- **"The Complete Guide to Aromatherapy" by Salvatore Battaglia**: This book is a thorough resource for both beginners and advanced practitioners. It covers essential oil profiles, therapeutic uses, and blending techniques, making it an excellent guide for creating your own aromatherapy products.
- **"The Art of Aromatherapy" by Robert Tisserand**: Written by one of the foremost experts in the field, this book is a classic that offers detailed information on the therapeutic properties of essential oils and their historical uses.
- **"Aromatherapy for the Soul" by Valerie Ann Worwood**: This book explores the emotional and spiritual benefits of aromatherapy, offering guidance on how to use essential oils for emotional healing, meditation, and personal growth.

Online Courses and Certifications

For those looking to dive deeper into aromatherapy with structured learning, online courses and certifications provide valuable, practical education. These courses often include video tutorials, lectures, and hands-on activities to develop your skills in blending, safety protocols, and therapeutic practices.

- **The Aromahead Institute** offers a variety of online courses, ranging from beginner to advanced levels. Their programs include certification courses in aromatherapy, essential oils, and blending, helping students gain practical knowledge while earning recognized credentials.
- **National Association for Holistic Aromatherapy (NAHA)** provides certification programs that focus on the safe and professional use of essential oils. Their

educational materials include detailed content on how to use aromatherapy for health and wellness.
- **The Tisserand Institute** offers a range of online courses that are designed for both professionals and those interested in learning aromatherapy for personal use. Robert Tisserand's expertise guides students through topics like essential oil safety, blending techniques, and the science behind aromatherapy.

Websites and Blogs

Staying updated with the latest trends, research, and practical advice on aromatherapy is easy thanks to the many online resources. Many well-known aromatherapists and essential oil companies maintain websites and blogs that offer free tips, articles, and product recommendations.

- **AromaWeb**: This is an excellent online resource for aromatherapy enthusiasts. It includes essential oil profiles, blending guides, and articles on the safe and effective use of essential oils. AromaWeb is a great place to explore the science behind essential oils, along with practical tips for daily use.
- **The Tisserand Institute Blog**: Robert Tisserand's blog provides insightful articles on essential oil safety, new research, and best practices for using oils therapeutically. His work is widely respected in the aromatherapy community and is a valuable resource for anyone looking to deepen their knowledge.
- **Edens Garden Blog**: As a major supplier of essential oils, Edens Garden offers a blog with practical advice on aromatherapy use, DIY recipes, and information about the therapeutic benefits of different oils. They also provide a range of free educational materials for their customers.

Workshops and Conferences

Attending workshops and conferences allows aromatherapy practitioners to learn from industry experts and network with like-minded individuals. These events offer hands-on learning and opportunities to deepen your practice in a supportive environment.

- **NAHA Conferences**: The National Association for Holistic Aromatherapy hosts annual conferences and workshops that offer continuing education for both professionals and enthusiasts. These events feature expert speakers, practical demonstrations, and the latest in aromatherapy research and techniques.
- **Aromatherapy International Events**: Many international organizations and schools host workshops, webinars, and retreats to help you stay informed and engaged with the global aromatherapy community. Attending these events provides opportunities to learn from world-renowned aromatherapists and essential oil experts.

Podcasts and YouTube Channels

For those looking to absorb knowledge on the go, podcasts and YouTube channels are great alternatives. These resources allow you to learn while commuting, exercising, or relaxing.

- **The Aromatherapy Podcast**: Hosted by various aromatherapy experts, this podcast covers a wide range of topics, from blending essential oils to using aromatherapy for specific health concerns. The podcast offers an accessible way learn more about the art and science of aromatherapy.
- **Aromahead Institute YouTube Channel**: The Aromahead Institute provides educational videos on essential oils, blending, and aromatherapy safety. Their YouTube channel is an excellent way to watch demonstrations and gain practica knowledge from certified professionals.
- **The Essential Oil Revolution**: This podcast offers expert interviews, tips, and personal stories from successful aromatherapists. It covers essential oil safety, business advice for aromatherapy practitioners, and product development tips.

Social Media Communities and Forums

Joining online communities dedicated to aromatherapy allows you to connect with othe share experiences, and ask questions. These spaces are great for staying motivated, finding inspiration, and learning new techniques.

- **Facebook Groups**: Many Facebook groups are dedicated to aromatherapy, whe members can share personal experiences, tips, and product recommendations. Groups like "Aromatherapy and Essential Oils" or "Essential Oils for Health an Wellness" are popular places to ask questions and exchange ideas.
- **Reddit**: Subreddits like r/Aromatherapy or r/essentialoils are active communitie where users discuss the latest trends, share personal experiences, and provide advice on using essential oils for health and wellness.
- **Instagram**: Instagram is filled with aromatherapy practitioners, enthusiasts, and companies sharing tips, product demos, and essential oil recipes. By following hashtags like #Aromatherapy, #EssentialOils, or #NaturalHealing, you can discover new content and connect with professionals.

Local Aromatherapy Practitioners

If you prefer more personalized, hands-on learning, consider seeking out local aromatherapists or wellness centers that offer workshops, private consultations, or grou classes. Many practitioners host sessions to teach blending techniques, the safe use of essential oils, or how to incorporate aromatherapy into daily life.

Conclusion

With so many resources available, expanding your aromatherapy knowledge has never been easier. From books and online courses to podcasts, workshops, and community forums, there is an abundance of opportunities to deepen your understanding and skills. As you continue your journey into the world of aromatherapy, these resources can help you build confidence, enhance your well-being, and create a more fulfilling, holistic lifestyle.

Building a Career in Aromatherapy

Building a career in aromatherapy offers a rewarding path for those interested in holistic health and wellness. As more people seek natural remedies for physical, emotional, and mental well-being, aromatherapy has become an increasingly popular field. Whether you're looking to become an aromatherapy practitioner, educator, product maker, or consultant, there are multiple avenues to explore. By gaining the right knowledge, certifications, and experience, you can turn your passion for essential oils and holistic healing into a fulfilling profession.

1. Education and Certification

One of the first steps to establishing a career in aromatherapy is obtaining proper education and certification. While there is no universal certification requirement, recognized programs help ensure you are knowledgeable about essential oils, safety practices, and therapeutic applications.

- **Formal Training**: Accredited schools and institutes offer courses in aromatherapy, ranging from basic workshops to comprehensive diploma or certification programs. Look for programs that are recognized by professional bodies such as the **National Association for Holistic Aromatherapy (NAHA)** or the **Aromatherapy Trade Council (ATC)**. These certifications validate your expertise and demonstrate professionalism to potential clients or employers.
- **Specialized Areas**: You may also choose to specialize in areas like **aromatherapy for pain management**, **stress relief**, **skin care**, or **emotional healing**. Continuing education in these areas will make you stand out in specific markets, whether you're working in clinical settings, spas, or wellness centers.
- **Hands-on Practice**: Many aromatherapy courses offer practical experience, where you'll get to practice creating blends, using essential oils, and working with clients. This hands-on experience is crucial in honing your skills and understanding how essential oils interact with the body.

2. Gaining Experience

Once you've acquired the necessary education and certification, gaining practical experience is essential. Building a career in aromatherapy relies on working directly with clients, whether through one-on-one consultations, group workshops, or hands-on treatments.

- **Volunteer or Intern**: Seek opportunities to work with experienced practitioners or at wellness centers, spas, or natural health stores. Interning or volunteering allows you to observe seasoned professionals, ask questions, and refine your skills in a real-world environment.
- **Freelance and Build a Client Base**: Starting your own practice or working as a freelance aromatherapist gives you the flexibility to work with clients in various settings, including their homes, wellness clinics, or corporate offices. Word of mouth and social media can help build your reputation, allowing you to grow your client base over time.
- **Working in Spas or Wellness Centers**: Many spas and holistic wellness centers are adding aromatherapy services to their menus. Working as an aromatherapist at a spa gives you the opportunity to gain experience with a wide range of clients, offering treatments such as massages, facials, or personalized aromatherapy sessions.

Developing Specialties

As the field of aromatherapy continues to expand, there are increasing opportunities to carve out a niche or specialty that sets you apart. Specializing in certain areas allows you to become an expert in specific applications of aromatherapy, making you more appealing to certain target audiences.

- **Aromatherapy for Mental Health**: With growing awareness around mental health, aromatherapy has become a valuable tool for addressing stress, anxiety, depression, and other emotional concerns. Specializing in aromatherapy for emotional well-being can open doors to work in clinical settings or as part of a therapy team.
- **Aromatherapy for Skin Care**: Natural beauty and skincare products infused with essential oils are in high demand. Specializing in creating skincare products or providing aromatherapy facials can be a lucrative and fulfilling aspect of your career.
- **Aromatherapy for Pregnancy and Children**: There is a growing demand for aromatherapy services tailored to the unique needs of pregnant women and children. Ensuring that you have the proper knowledge and training in these areas will allow you to offer safe and effective treatments to these sensitive populations.

Starting Your Own Aromatherapy Business

Another pathway to building a successful career in aromatherapy is to start your own business. Aromatherapy is a versatile field that offers various business opportunities, from creating essential oil products to offering consultation services.

- **Product Development**: You can create and sell your own line of essential oils, aromatherapy blends, bath products, candles, or skincare items. Building a brand around natural and therapeutic products can help you tap into the growing demand for organic and wellness-focused products. Establishing an online store or partnering with retail outlets or wellness centers can help reach a wider audience.
- **Workshops and Classes**: Offering workshops, seminars, or online courses about aromatherapy can be a rewarding way to share your knowledge with others. Teaching others how to use essential oils safely and effectively for various purposes can establish you as an expert in the field and provide a valuable income stream.
- **Consultation and Coaching**: If you have a strong background in aromatherapy and wellness, you could offer one-on-one coaching or consultation services. This could include helping clients incorporate aromatherapy into their daily lives, advising businesses on using essential oils in their offerings, or providing corporate wellness programs focused on aromatherapy for stress reduction and productivity.

5. Marketing and Networking

To build a career in aromatherapy, effective marketing and networking are key to growing your visibility and connecting with potential clients. As with any business, developing a strong personal or professional brand can help you stand out in a competitive market.

- **Online Presence**: Having a website and active social media profiles is essential for showcasing your expertise, sharing client testimonials, and offering tips or educational content related to aromatherapy. Platforms like Instagram, Pinterest, and Facebook are perfect for visually showcasing your products or services, while LinkedIn can help you connect with potential business collaborators.
- **Networking**: Attend aromatherapy conferences, wellness expos, and community events to connect with other professionals in the field. Networking with health practitioners, spas, wellness centers, and even medical professionals can lead to valuable collaborations or client referrals.
- **Client Reviews**: Client testimonials and word-of-mouth recommendations are powerful tools in building trust and credibility. Encourage clients to leave reviews on your website or social media pages, which can help establish your reputation and attract new customers.

6. Staying Informed and Continuing Education

The field of aromatherapy is constantly evolving, with new research and practices emerging regularly. To stay competitive, it's important to continue learning and adapting to changes in the industry.

- **Conferences and Workshops**: Attend aromatherapy and wellness conferences to stay informed about new trends, products, and research. These events are great opportunities for professional development and networking.
- **Certifications**: Consider pursuing advanced certifications in areas like clinical aromatherapy, product formulation, or specific modalities like aromatherapy for emotional well-being. Continuing education can deepen your expertise and broaden your career opportunities.
- **Read Industry Publications**: Subscribe to aromatherapy journals, blogs, and newsletters to keep up with the latest research, product developments, and industry news.

Conclusion

Building a career in aromatherapy offers diverse opportunities in a rapidly growing field. Whether you're interested in providing hands-on treatments, creating your own products, or educating others, there are multiple paths to success. With proper training, experience, and dedication, you can establish a rewarding and sustainable career in this holistic, healing profession. By continuing to expand your knowledge, refine your skills, and connect with the community, you can make a meaningful impact on the lives of others while fostering your own personal growth.

Have Questions / Comments?

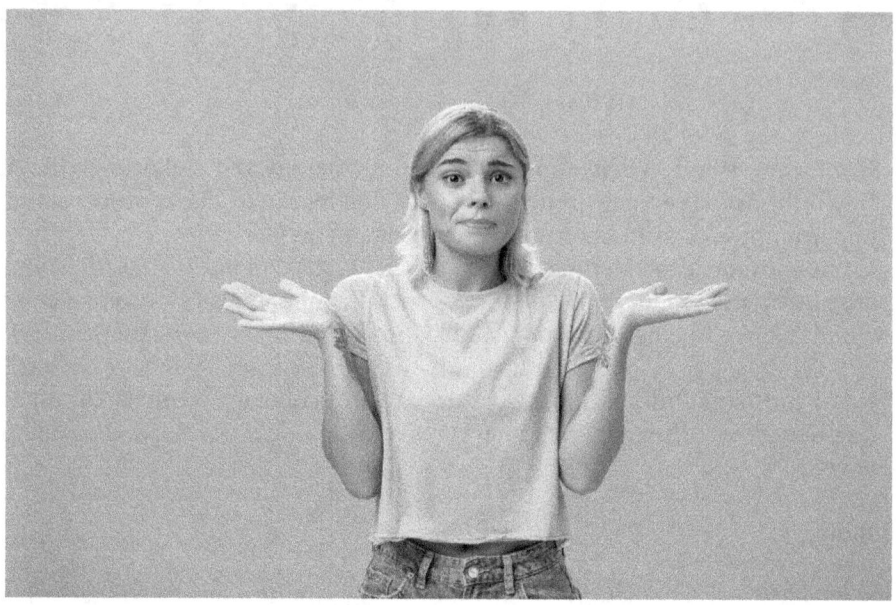

This book was designed to cover as much as possible but I know I have probably missed something, or some new amazing discovery that has just come out.

If you notice something missing or have a question that I failed to answer, please get in touch and let me know. If I can, I will email you an answer and also update the book so others can also benefit from it.

Thanks For Being Awesome :)

Submit Your Questions / Comments At:

https://questions.xspurts.com

Get Another Book Free

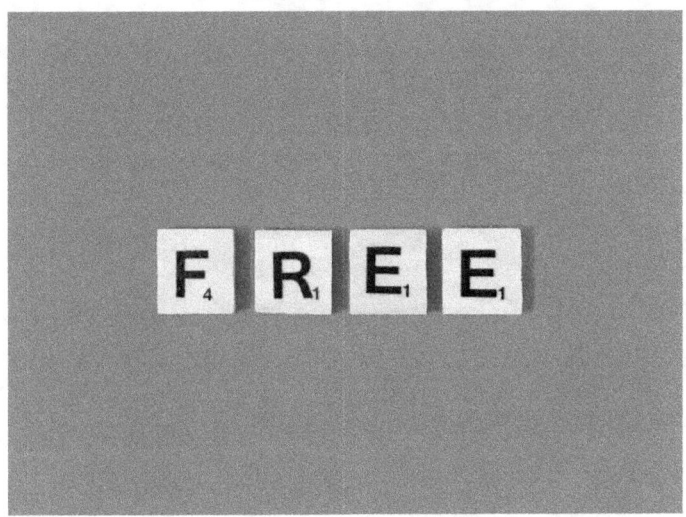

We love writing and have produced a huge number of books.

For being one of our amazing readers, we would love to offer you another book we have created, 100% free.

To claim this limited time special offer, simply go to the site below and enter your name and email address.

You will then receive one of my great books, direct to your email account, 100% free!

https://free.xspurts.com

www.ingramcontent.com/pod-product-compliance
Lightning Source LLC
Chambersburg PA
CBHW071056240526
45471CB00016B/1970